QUICK [illegible]

MISSION OF THE AMERICAN RED CROSS

The American Red Cross, a humanitarian organization led by volunteers and guided by its Congressional Charter and the Fundamental Principles of the International Red Cross Movement, will provide relief to victims of disasters and help people prevent, prepare for, and respond to emergencies.

PRINCIPLES OF THE INTERNATIONAL RED CROSS

Humanity
Impartiality
Neutrality
Independence
Voluntary Service
Unity
Universality

www.redcross.org

American Red Cross

AMERICAN RED CROSS
FIRST AID FAST

First Aid Fast is intended to give you the basic information you need to effectively respond to an emergency. *This book is not a substitute for training!* An American Red Cross course gives you an opportunity to learn and practice life-saving skills and allows you to have all of your questions answered by a knowledgeable instructor. *First Aid Fast* should be your first step — not your only step — toward becoming a valuable first aider.

This booklet is not intended to replace current manuals being used in American Red Cross courses resulting in First Aid or CPR certification. Only courses conducted by American Red Cross certified instructors in accordance with American Red Cross policies and procedures are considered formal American Red Cross training.

StayWell®

StayWell®

This book, by itself, does not constitute complete and comprehensive training.

The emergency care procedures outlined in this book reflect the standard of knowledge and accepted emergency practices in the United States at the time this book was published. It is the reader's responsibility to stay informed of changes in the emergency care procedures.

The Care Steps for CPR outlined within this product are consistent with the Guidelines 2000 for Cardiopulmonary Resuscitation and Emergency Cardiovascular Care.

Printed in the United States of America.

StayWell®
780 Township Line Road
Yardley, PA 19067

ISBN 1-58480-130-1

03 04 05 06 / 9 8 7 6 5 4 3 2

HOW TO USE THIS BOOK

First Aid Fast can be used two ways. First, it can be read to help familiarize yourself with the emergencies that can happen wherever you may be — home, workplace, school, or vacation. By looking at the book before an emergency, you can be better prepared to react. Second, it provides a quick source of information in emergencies. Each section guides your actions, step-by-step.

ORGANIZATION

A Quick Reference — that provides an alphabetical listing of signals and conditions — can be found at the front of this book. The Quick Reference is designed to get you to the care you need quickly. For example, if someone at your dinner table begins choking, search for "Choking." If someone is experiencing pain or pressure in the chest, look up "Chest pain."

HOW TO USE THIS BOOK

DESIGN

Information and step-by-step actions for problems requiring first aid are presented both as text and pictures. Signals are listed first. A list of care steps follows. Pictures have been included where they are most helpful.

USAGE

***First Aid Fast* needs to be everywhere an accident or emergency could happen. Keep one in:**

- Home pool areas
- First aid kits (home and workplace)
- Automobile glove compartments
- Backpacks
- Briefcases

***First Aid Fast* is a thoughtful gift for:**

- Parents
- Babysitters or caregivers
- Teachers
- Scout leaders
- Coaches
- Neighbors

This booklet is not a substitute for materials used in American Red Cross courses in which First Aid or CPR certification is given.

AMERICAN RED CROSS
HEALTH AND SAFETY PROGRAMS

The American Red Cross offers a variety of community programs, some of which are available in Spanish, that teach life-saving skills and safety information. Contact your local American Red Cross for information on these and other programs.

American Red Cross Adult CPR
American Red Cross Community CPR
American Red Cross Community First Aid and Safety
American Red Cross Sport Safety Training
American Red Cross First Aid for Children Today (FACT)
American Red Cross Infant & Child CPR
American Red Cross Workplace Training: Standard First Aid
American Red Cross Adult CPR/AED
American Red Cross Basic Aid Training (for children)
American Red Cross Babysitter's Training
American Red Cross Community Water Safety
American Red Cross Learn to Swim Programs
American Red Cross GuardStart: Lifeguarding Tomorrow
American Red Cross Longfellow's Whale Tales (for children)
American Red Cross HIV/AIDS Programs

You can make a difference by presenting life-saving information in your community. Contact your local American Red Cross for more information about instructor training.

RESPONDING TO EMERGENCIES

Despite best efforts, emergencies can occur any place or time. In fact, at some time in your life, it is likely that you will witness a situation in which someone you know will require first aid...THAT SOMEONE MIGHT BE YOU!

Your community's emergency medical services (EMS) system depends on people like you to recognize and respond to emergencies for it to work effectively. This requires that you be able to:

- Recognize that an emergency exists
- Decide to act
- Call 9-1-1 or the local emergency number
- Provide care until help arrives

This booklet is not a substitute for materials used in American Red Cross courses in which First Aid or CPR certification is given.

HOW WILL I KNOW —
IF SOMEONE NEEDS MY HELP

Your senses — **hearing, sight, and smell** — may help you recognize an emergency. Emergencies are often signaled by something unusual that catches your attention.

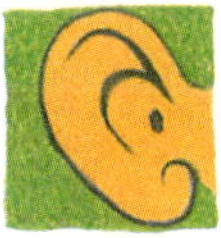
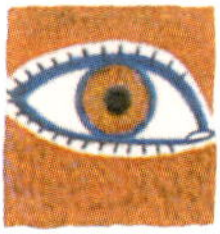
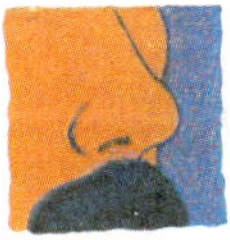
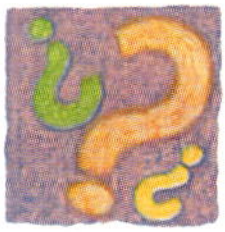

UNUSUAL NOISES

- Screams, yells, moans, or calls for help
- Breaking glass, crashing metal, or screeching tires
- Changes in machinery or equipment noises
- Sudden, loud voices

UNUSUAL SIGHTS

- A stalled vehicle
- An overturned pot
- A spilled medicine container
- Broken glass
- Downed electrical wires
- Smoke or fire

UNUSUAL ODORS

- Strong or unrecognizable odors

UNUSUAL APPEARANCES OR BEHAVIOR

- Trouble breathing
- Clutching the chest or throat
- Slurred or confused speech
- Unexplainable confusion or drowsiness
- Sweating for no apparent reason
- Unusual skin color

EMERGENCY ACTION STEPS

In the excitement of an emergency, you may be frightened or confused about what to do. STAY CALM — you can help. An emergency scene might look complicated at first but the three EMERGENCY ACTION STEPS will help you organize your response to the situation.

1	CHECK	*Check the scene and the victim.*
2	CALL	*Call 9-1-1 or your local emergency number.*
3	CARE	*Care for the victim.*

This booklet is not a substitute for materials used in American Red Cross courses in which First Aid or CPR certification is given.

HOW AND WHEN TO CALL 9-1-1

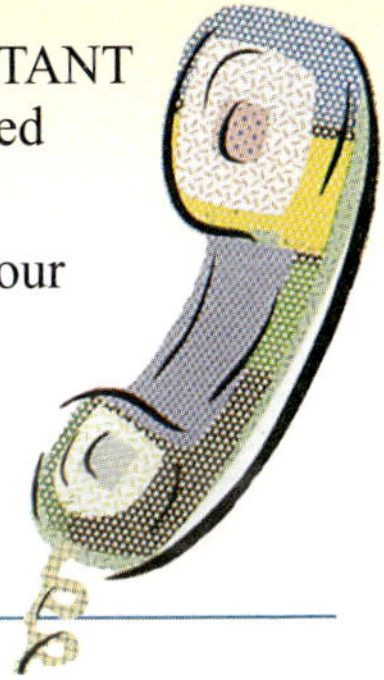

Calling for help is often the MOST IMPORTANT action you can take to help the person in need of aid.

If the person is unconscious, call 9-1-1 or your local emergency number immediately.

Sometimes a conscious person will tell you not to call 9-1-1, and you may not be sure what to do.

Call anyway if the person:

- Is or becomes unconscious
- Has trouble breathing or is breathing in a strange way
- Has chest pain or pressure
- Is bleeding severely
- Has pressure or pain in the abdomen that does not go away
- Is vomiting or passing blood
- Has seizures, a severe headache, or slurred speech
- Appears to have been poisoned
- Has injuries to the head, neck, or back
- Has possible broken bones

Also call for any of these situations:

- Fire or explosion
- Downed electrical wires
- Swiftly moving or rapidly rising water
- Presence of poisonous gas
- Vehicle collisions
- Persons who cannot be moved easily

HOW AND WHEN TO CALL 9-1-1

WHEN YOU ARE ALONE

Call First, that is, call 9-1-1 or the local emergency number before providing care for:

- An unconscious adult or child 8 years old or older
- An unconscious infant or child known to be at high risk for heart problems

Call First situations are likely to be cardiac emergencies, such as sudden cardiac arrest, where *time is critical.*

Call Fast, that is, provide 1 minute of care, then call 9-1-1 or the local emergency number for:

- An unconscious victim less than 8 years old
- Any victim of submersion or near drowning
- Any victim of cardiac arrest associated with trauma
- Any victim of drug overdose

Call Fast situations are likely to be related to breathing emergencies, rather than sudden cardiac arrest. In these situations, provide support for airway, breathing, and circulation through rescue breaths or chest compressions as appropriate.

This booklet is not a substitute for materials used in American Red Cross courses in which First Aid or CPR certification is given.

WHAT YOU SHOULD KNOW ABOUT —

GOOD SAMARITAN LAWS

Good Samaritan laws were developed to encourage people to help others in emergency situations. These laws give legal protection to people who provide emergency care to ill or injured persons. They require that the "Good Samaritan" use common sense and a reasonable level of skill, not to go beyond the individual's level of training in emergency situations. They assume each person would do his or her best to save a life or prevent further injury.

If you are interested in finding out about your state's Good Samaritan laws, contact a legal professional or your state attorney general's office, or check with your local library.

Remember to get consent (the victim accepts your offer to help) before caring for a conscious victim. For an unconscious victim, consent is implied.

WHAT YOU SHOULD KNOW ABOUT —

PREVENTING DISEASE TRANSMISSION

By following some basic guidelines, you can help to reduce disease transmission when providing first aid:

- Avoid contact with body fluids, such as blood, when possible
- Place barriers, such as disposable gloves or a clean dry cloth, between the victim's body fluids and yourself
- Cover any cuts, scrapes, and openings in your skin by wearing protective clothing, such as disposable gloves
- Use breathing barriers, if available, when breathing for a person
- Wash your hands with soap and water immediately before and after giving care, even if you wear gloves
- Do not eat, drink, or touch your mouth, nose, or eyes when giving first aid
- Do not touch objects that may be soiled with blood, mucus, or other body substances

Following these guidelines decreases your risk of getting or transmitting diseases. Remember always to give first aid in ways that protect you and the victim from disease transmission. The American Red Cross recommends the use of a breathing barrier when performing CPR or rescue breaths if you are concerned about making direct contact with a victim.

This booklet is not a substitute for materials used in American Red Cross courses in which First Aid or CPR certification is given.

BREATHING EMERGENCIES —

NOT BREATHING (UNCONSCIOUS)

SIGNALS

- Chest does not rise and fall
- Can't feel or hear breaths
- Skin appears pale or bluish

CARE

- CHECK the scene and the victim
- Send someone to CALL 9-1-1 or the local emergency number
- Tilt head back and lift chin
- Look, listen, and feel for breathing for about 5 seconds

If person is not breathing:

- Pinch person's nose shut, open your mouth wide, and make a tight seal around the person's mouth. (For infant, cover both mouth and nose with your mouth)
- Give 2 slow breaths, until the chest clearly rises
- Check for movement (coughing or response to breaths) for about 10 seconds

If the victim is breathing but remains unconscious:

- Place the victim on his/her side in case he or she vomits, and monitor breathing and movement

If the victim is not breathing but shows some movement (coughing or response to breaths):

- Perform rescue breathing
  Adult: Give 1 slow rescue breath about every 5 seconds
  Child or infant: Give 1 slow rescue breath about every 3 seconds
- Recheck for breathing and movement about every minute

BREATHING EMERGENCIES —

RESCUE BREATHING

1

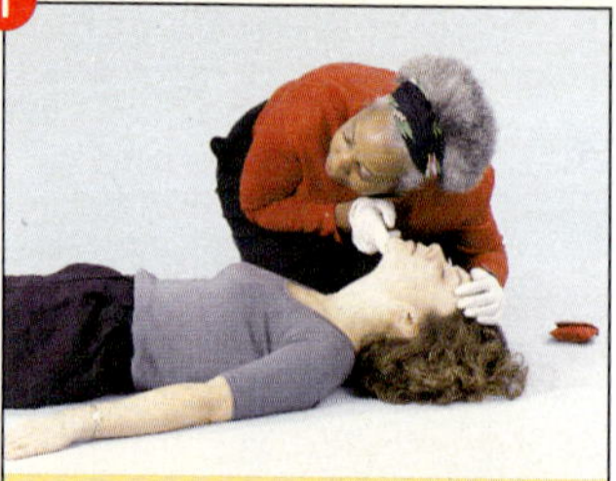

- Tilt the head back and lift the chin to open the airway

2

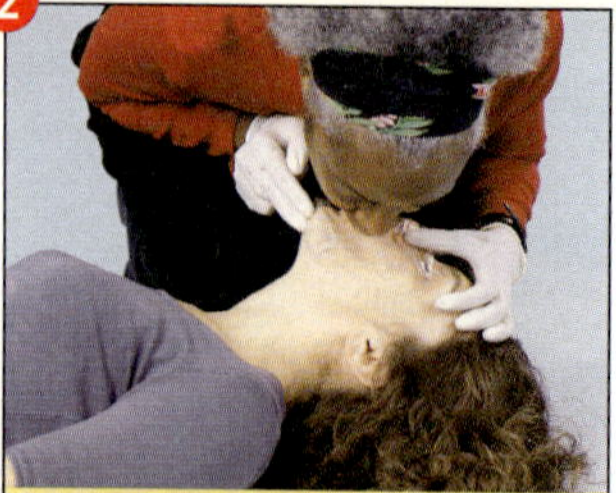

ADULT:

- Give 1 slow breath about every 5 seconds

3

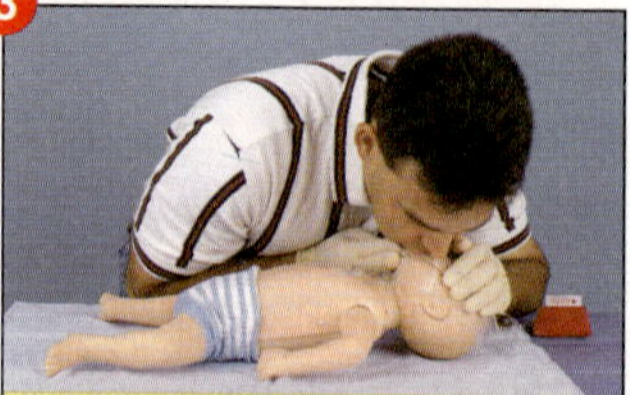

CHILD/INFANT:

- Give 1 slow breath about every 3 seconds

- Recheck breathing and movement. If no movement, begin CPR (see Cardiac Emergencies — pp. 25-29)

This booklet is not a substitute for materials used in American Red Cross courses in which First Aid or CPR certification is given.

BREATHING EMERGENCIES —
SPECIAL SITUATIONS

HEAD, NECK, OR BACK INJURY

Head, neck, or back injuries may result from a fall from a height, an automobile collision, or a diving accident. Use the jaw-thrust maneuver when checking breathing and giving breaths:

- Place one hand on each side of the victim's head with your thumbs on the victim's cheeks and your fingers under the back of the lower jaw, next to the ears
- Grab the back of the lower jaw, next to the the ears, and lift with both hands
- If you can maintain a clear, open airway, do not move the victim unnecessarily
- If you give rescue breaths, place your cheek tightly against the victim's nose

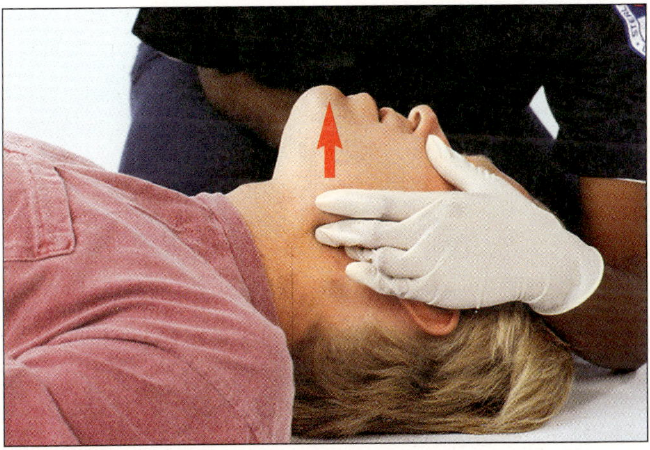

BREATHING EMERGENCIES —
SPECIAL SITUATIONS

DROWNING

Drownings often happen to persons who never intended to get wet. Drownings can also happen in the home in as little water as a bucketful.

- Send someone to CALL 9-1-1 or the local emergency number

Once the person is out of the water:

- CHECK the person, CARE for any conditions you find
- Tilt the head back and CHECK breathing. CHECK the mouth for fluid or objects

If airway appears clear:

- Give 2 slow rescue breaths

If breaths do not go in:

- Reposition the airway and reattempt breaths

If breaths still do not go in:

- See Choking — Unconscious (pp. 32-35)

BREATHING EMERGENCIES —

SPECIAL SITUATIONS

NECK BREATHER (STOMA)

A person who has had part or all of the voice box removed breathes through a hole in the throat (called a stoma) instead of the mouth and nose. There may be visible scarring at the base of the neck. This person may wear a medical alert identification.

- CHECK for breathing at the stoma
- When giving rescue breaths, breathe into the stoma in the same way you would give breaths at the mouth

BURNS

Burns are caused by heat, chemicals, electricity, and radiation. The severity of a burn depends on the temperature of whatever caused the burn, the length of time the person is exposed, the location on the body, the burn's size, and the person's age and medical condition.

SIGNALS

SUPERFICIAL BURNS

- The skin is red and dry
- Area may swell and is usually painful

DEEP BURNS

- The skin is red and has blisters that may open and weep clear fluid
- Area may swell and is usually painful
- May appear brown or black
- Can range from very painful to almost painless

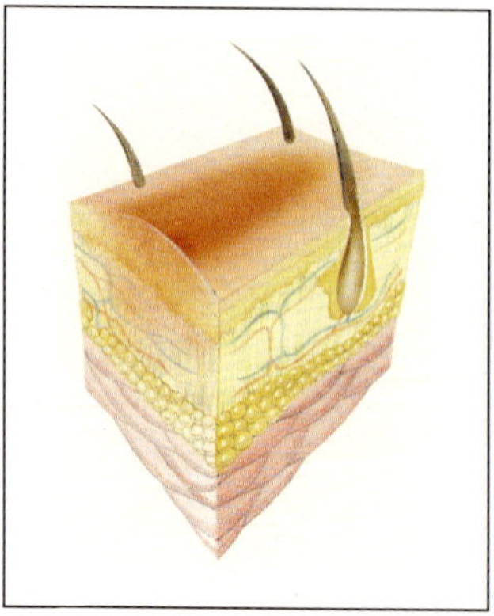

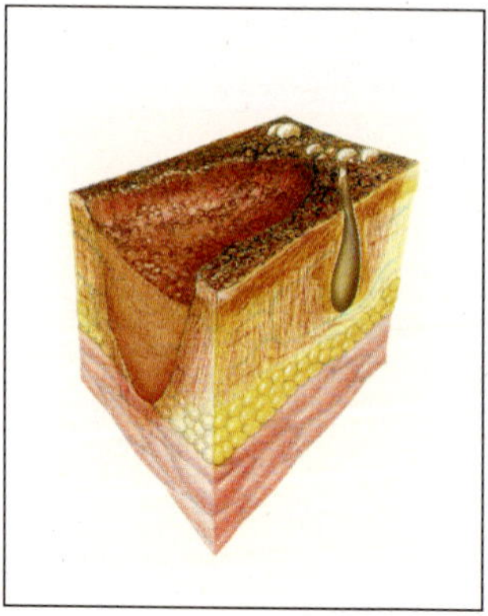

This booklet is not a substitute for materials used in American Red Cross courses in which First Aid or CPR certification is given.

BURNS

CARE

- CHECK the scene and the victim
- Send someone to CALL 9-1-1 or the local emergency number
- Stop the burning. Remove person from source of the burn
- Cool the burn. Use large amounts of cool water. Do not use ice or ice water except on small superficial burns. Apply soaked towels, sheets, or other wet cloth to the face or other areas that cannot be immersed. Keep cloth cool by adding more water
- Cover the burn. Use dry, sterile dressings or a clean cloth. Loosely bandage dressing in place to prevent infection and reduce pain, or cover burned area with dry sheet
- Keep the victim from getting chilled or overheated

WHEN TO CALL 9-1-1 OR THE LOCAL EMERGENCY NUMBER

- Burns involving trouble breathing
- Burns covering more than one body part
- Burns to the head, neck, hands, feet, or genitals
- Burns (other than a very minor one) to a child or elderly person
- Burns resulting from chemicals, explosions, or electricity

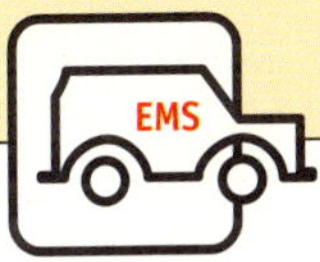

BURNS

1

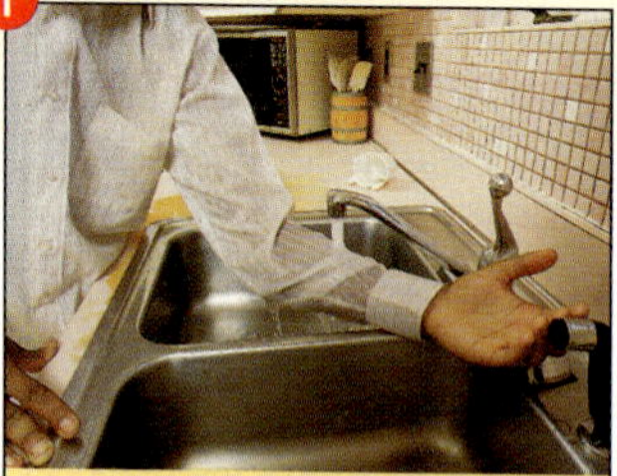

- Stop the burning

2

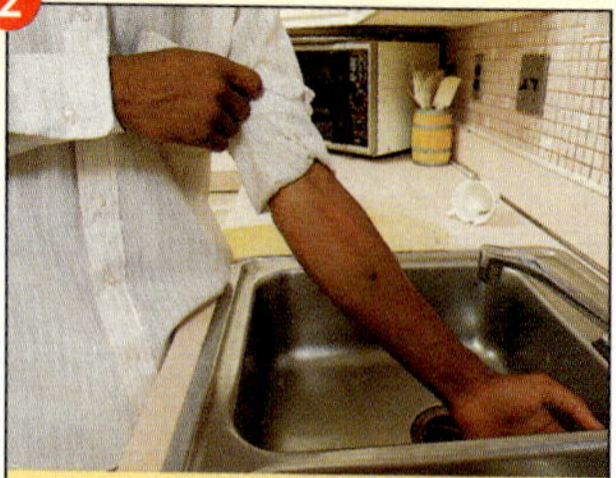

- Cool the burned area with large amounts of cool water

3

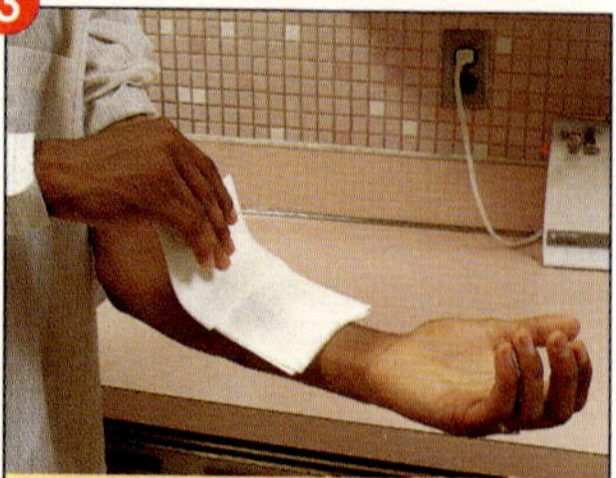

- Cover the burn with dry, clean dressings or cloth

This booklet is not a substitute for materials used in American Red Cross courses in which First Aid or CPR certification is given.

BURNS —
SPECIAL SITUATIONS

SUNBURN

- Cool the burn
- Protect from further damage by staying out of sun or wearing sunscreen
- Protect unbroken blisters with loose bandages and keep broken blisters clean to prevent infection

ELECTRICAL BURNS

- CHECK the scene and the victim
- Send someone to CALL 9-1-1 or the local emergency number
- Never go near a victim until the power is turned off. If a power line is down, wait for the fire department or power company
- If victim is unconscious, give rescue breathing (see Breathing Emergencies — p. 12) or CPR (see Cardiac Emergencies — pp. 25-29) if needed
- Do not move victim unnecessarily because there may be internal injuries
- CHECK for possibility of two wounds: entrance and exit burns
- Do not cool burn
- Cover burn with dry, sterile dressing
- Keep the victim from getting chilled or overheated

BURNS — SPECIAL SITUATIONS

CHEMICAL BURNS

- CHECK the scene to make sure it is safe
- Send someone to CALL 9-1-1 or the local emergency number, if necessary
- For a wet chemical, flush affected areas with large amounts of cool running water until ambulance arrives. Always flush away from the body. Brush dry chemicals off the skin with a gloved hand
- Remove clothing and jewelry that may trap chemicals against the skin or on which chemicals may have spilled

SMOKE INHALATION

- Move the person to fresh air
- Send someone to CALL 9-1-1 or the local emergency number
- If the victim is unconscious, give rescue breathing (see Breathing Emergencies — p. 12) or CPR (see Cardiac Emergencies — pp. 25-29) if needed
- Support the person in the position in which it is easiest to breathe
- If person is breathing but unconscious, place on side and monitor breathing closely

CARDIAC (HEART) EMERGENCIES

There are two general types of cardiac emergencies — when the heart doesn't function properly, depriving the heart muscle of much needed oxygen and causing chest pain or discomfort (heart attack) and when the heart doesn't function at all (cardiac arrest).

Cardiac Chain of Survival

The greatest chance of survival from cardiac arrest occurs when the following sequence of events happens as rapidly as possible:

1 Early recognition and early access.

The sooner 9-1-1 or the local emergency number is called, the sooner early advanced life support arrives.

2 Early CPR.

Early CPR helps circulate blood that contains oxygen to the vital organs until an AED is ready to use or emergency personnel arrive.

3 Early defibrillation.

Most victims of sudden cardiac arrest need an electric shock to the heart called defibrillation. Each minute that defibrillation is delayed reduces the chance of survival by about 10 percent.

4 Early advanced life support.

This is given by trained medical personnel who provide further care and transport to hospital facilities.

CARDIAC (HEART) EMERGENCIES

Sudden cardiac arrest claims the lives of 220,000 people in this country every year — almost one every 2 minutes. A quarter of these deaths can be prevented if an automated external defibrillator (AED) is available at the time of the emergency. An AED is a small, portable device that automatically analyzes a heart rhythm, and, if necessary, prompts a trained responder to deliver a life-saving shock to restore a heart's normal rhythm. Immediate use of an AED, in conjunction with CPR, could save up to 50,000 lives each year.

Ordinary people can be lifesavers, thanks to AEDs and training from your American Red Cross. AEDs are becoming more widely available and being used in a variety of settings, including airplanes and airports, office buildings, industrial plants, casinos, golf courses, cruise ships, sports arenas and health clubs. Does your community or place of employment have an AED and people who are trained to use it? Contact your local American Red Cross for more information on AEDs and AED training.

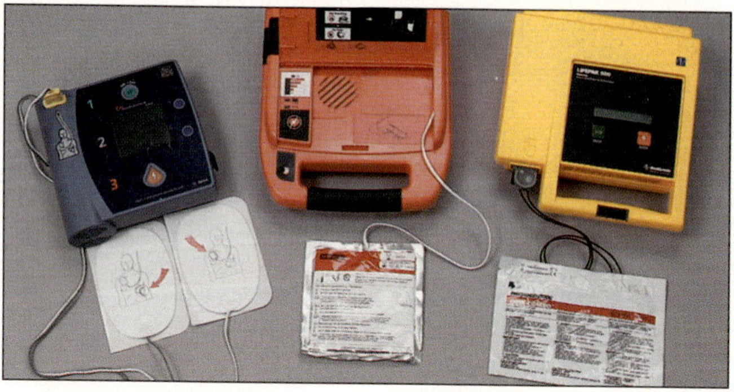

This booklet is not a substitute for materials used in American Red Cross courses in which First Aid or CPR certification is given.

CARDIAC (HEART) EMERGENCIES —

CHEST PAIN / DISCOMFORT

Most people who die of heart attacks die within 2 hours after the first signals appear. Many lives are lost because people deny they are having a heart attack and delay calling for help.

Recognizing the signals of a heart attack and calling 9-1-1 or the local emergency number before the heart stops are critical steps to saving lives.

SIGNALS

- Chest pain or discomfort lasting more than 3-5 minutes or that goes away and comes back. Pain is not relieved by rest, changing position, or medication. May spread to shoulder, arm, back, neck, or jaw
- Trouble breathing. Breathing is often faster than normal. Person feels short of breath
- Nausea
- Sweating or changes in skin appearance
- Dizziness or unconsciousness
- Ache, heartburn, or indigestion. These signals are more likely to occur in women, the elderly, and diabetics

CARE

- Have the person stop activity and rest
- Send someone to CALL 9-1-1 or the local emergency number
- Help the person rest in a comfortable position. A sitting position may make breathing easier
- Loosen restrictive clothing
- Assist with prescribed medication
- Monitor breathing and movement closely
- Be prepared to give CPR and use an AED if the person loses consciousness and shows no movement

CARDIAC EMERGENCIES —

CARDIAC ARREST (ADULT)

CPR is given to a person who is not breathing and shows no movement (coughing or response to breaths). CPR is a combination of chest compressions and rescue breathing.

SIGNALS

- Unresponsive (unconscious)
- Not breathing and no movement (coughing or response to breaths)

CARE

- CHECK the scene and the victim
- Send someone to CALL 9-1-1 or the local emergency number. If you are alone, call first, then provide care
- CHECK for breathing

If not breathing:

- Tilt head back, pinch nose, and give 2 slow rescue breaths. Each breath should make the chest clearly rise
- CHECK for movement (coughing or response to breaths)

If no movement, begin CPR.

- Find hand position in center of chest over breastbone
- Position shoulders over hands. Compress chest 15 times in about 10 seconds
- Give 2 slow breaths
- Do 3 more sets of 15 compressions and 2 breaths
- Recheck breathing and movement. If no movement, continue sets of 15 compressions and 2 breaths until the ambulance arrives

This booklet is not a substitute for materials used in American Red Cross courses in which First Aid or CPR certification is given.

CARDIAC EMERGENCIES —

CPR (ADULT)

1

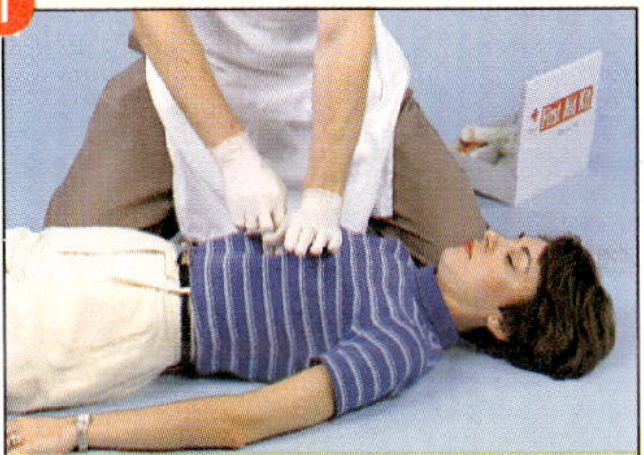

- Find hand position

2

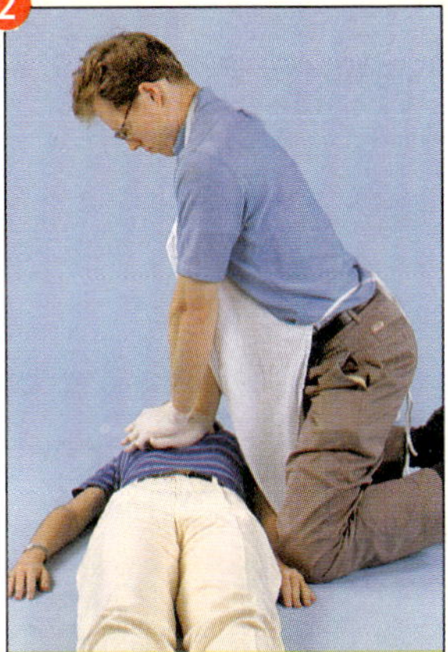

- Position shoulders over hands
- Compress chest 15 times

3

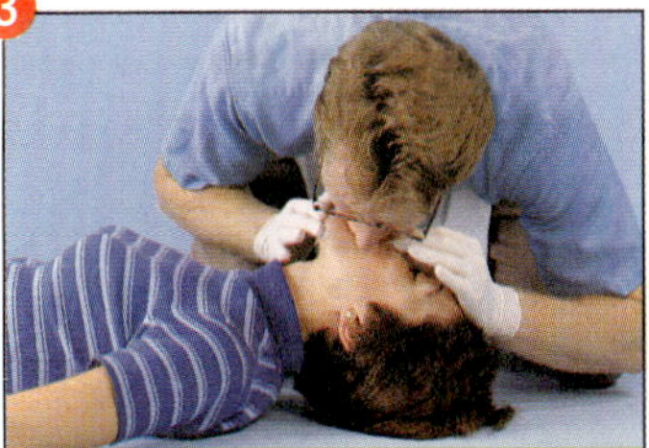

- Give 2 slow breaths
- Recheck breathing and movement. If no movement, continue sets of 15 compressions and 2 breaths

CARDIAC EMERGENCIES —
CARDIAC ARREST (CHILD)

When a child's heart stops, it is usually the result of a breathing emergency.

SIGNALS

- Unresponsive (unconscious)
- Not breathing and no movement (coughing or response to breaths)

CARE

- CHECK the scene and the child
- Send someone to CALL 9-1-1 or the local emergency number
- If you are alone, provide 1 minute of care before calling
- CHECK for breathing

If not breathing:

- Tilt head back, pinch nose, and give 2 slow rescue breaths. Each breath should make the chest clearly rise
- CHECK for movement (coughing or response to breaths)

If no movement, begin CPR.

- Find hand position in center of chest over breastbone
- Position shoulder over hand. Compress chest 5 times in about 3 seconds
- Give 1 slow breath
- Continue sets of 5 compressions and 1 breath for about a minute
- Recheck breathing and movement. If no movement, continue sets of 5 compressions and 1 breath until the ambulance arrives

CARDIAC EMERGENCIES —
CPR (CHILD)

1
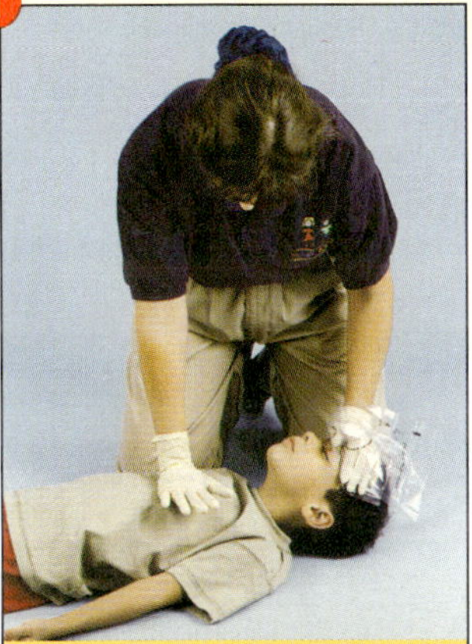

- Find hand position

2
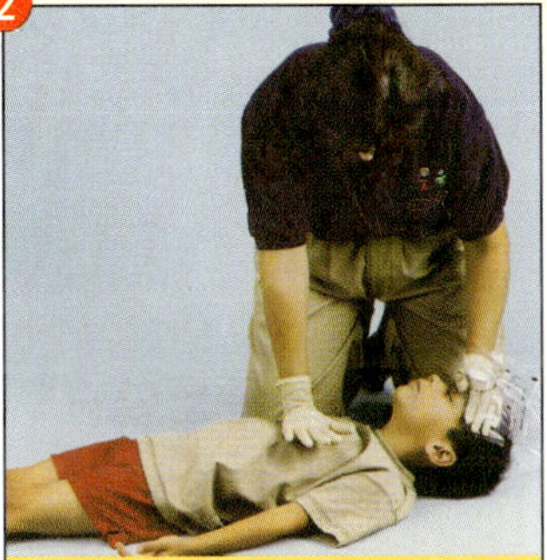

- Position shoulder over hand
- Compress chest 5 times

3
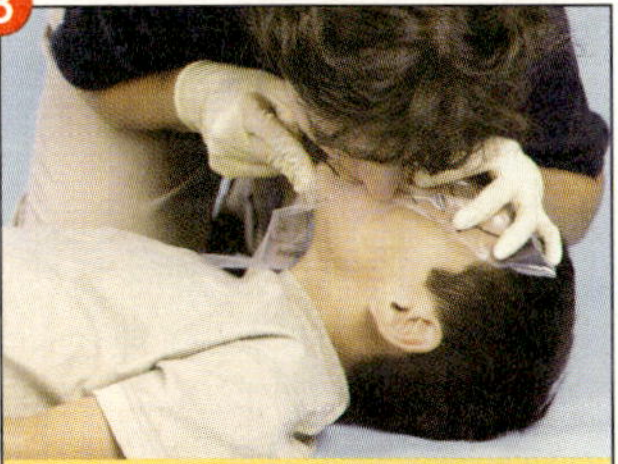

- Give 1 slow breath
- Recheck breathing and movement. If no movement, continue sets of 5 compressions and 1 breath

CARDIAC EMERGENCIES —

CARDIAC ARREST (INFANT)

When an infant's heart stops, it is usually the result of a breathing emergency.

SIGNALS

- Unresponsive (unconscious)
- Not breathing and no movement (coughing or response to breaths)

CARE

- CHECK the scene and the infant
- Send someone to CALL 9-1-1 or the local emergency number. If alone, provide 1 minute of care before calling
- CHECK for breathing

If not breathing:

- Tilt head back, cover mouth and nose, and give 2 slow rescue breaths. Each breath should make the chest clearly rise
- CHECK for movement (coughing or response to breaths)

If no movement, begin CPR.

- Find finger position in center of chest over breastbone
- Position hand over fingers. Compress chest 5 times in slightly less than 3 seconds
- Tilt head back, cover the infant's mouth and nose with your mouth, and give 1 slow breath
- Continue sets of 5 compressions and 1 breath for about a minute
- Recheck breathing and movement. If no movement, continue sets of 5 compressions and 1 breath until the ambulance arrives

CARDIAC EMERGENCIES —
CPR (INFANT)

1

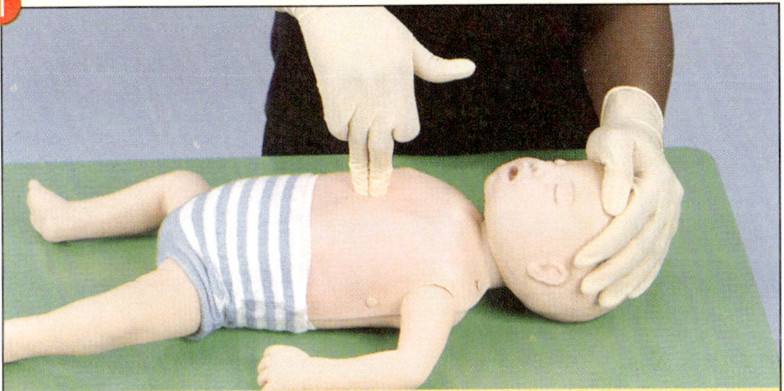

- Find finger position
- Position hand over fingers
- Compress chest 5 times

2

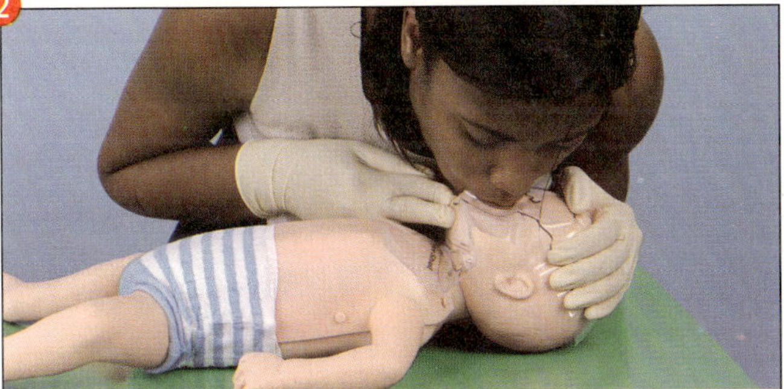

- Give 1 slow breath
- Recheck breathing and movement. If no movement, continue sets of 5 compressions and 1 breath

CHOKING —

CONSCIOUS ADULT AND CHILD

Although we think of choking as a common occurrence in children, more adults than children die each year as a result of choking. Common causes include trying to swallow large pieces of poorly chewed food; drinking alcohol before and during meals, dulling the nerves that aid in swallowing; eating while talking excitedly or laughing; eating too fast; and walking, playing, or running with food or objects in the mouth.

SIGNALS

- Clutching throat with one or both hands
- Unable to speak, cough forcefully, or breathe
- High-pitched wheezing

CARE

- CHECK the scene and the victim
- Send someone to CALL 9-1-1 or the local emergency number and get consent before providing care
- Place thumb side of fist against middle of abdomen just above the navel. Grasp fist with other hand
- Give quick, upward thrusts

Repeat until object is coughed up and person breathes on his or her own or person becomes unconscious.

If person becomes unconscious, look for an object in the mouth. If object is seen, remove it with your finger. Continue with care for Choking — Unconscious Adult (pp. 32-33) or Child (pp. 34-35).

CHOKING —
CONSCIOUS ADULT AND CHILD

1

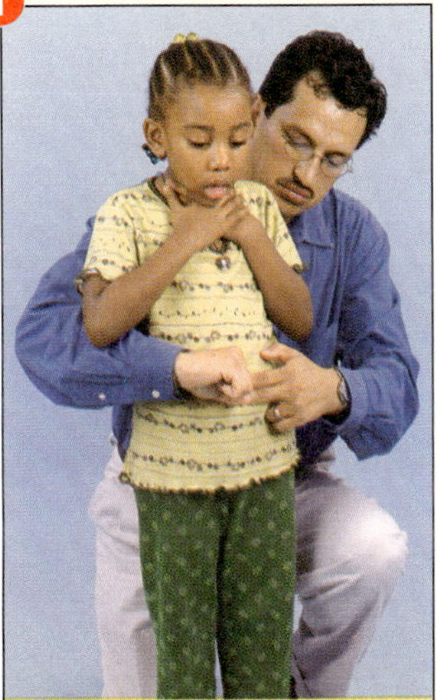

- Position hands

- For an adult, in most cases you will need to stand

2

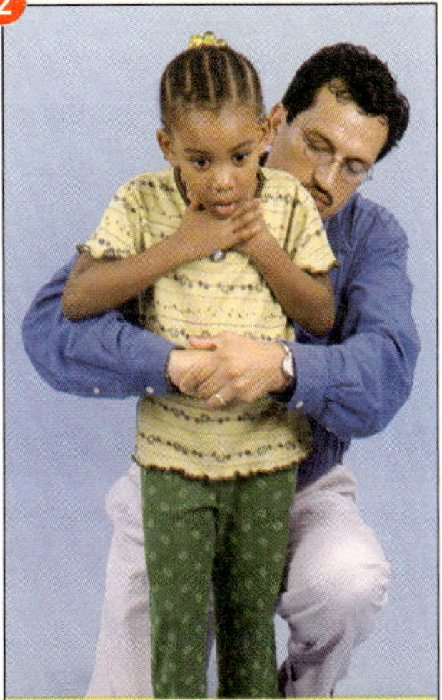

- Give quick, upward thrusts
- Repeat until object is coughed up and person breathes on own or person becomes unconscious

CHOKING —
UNCONSCIOUS ADULT

The airway can become blocked by the tongue falling back in the throat or by food, objects, or fluids — such as blood, saliva, or mucus — becoming lodged in the airway.

SIGNALS

- Unable to make the chest rise when giving rescue breaths

CARE

- Send someone to CALL 9-1-1 or the local emergency number. If alone, provide 1 minute of care before calling
- Tilt head back, lift chin, and pinch nose shut
- Give 2 slow rescue breaths. Breathe in until chest clearly rises
- If chest does not rise while giving breaths, REPOSITION airway and reattempt breaths

If breaths still do not go in:

- Find hand position in center of chest over breastbone
- Position shoulders over hands
- Compress chest 15 times in about 10 seconds
- Lift lower jaw and tongue and look for object in mouth. If object is visible, remove it with your index finger
- Tilt head back, lift chin, and pinch nose shut, and give 2 slow rescue breaths

If breaths still do not go in:

- Continue sets of 15 compressions, followed by look for object/removal and 2 rescue breaths until chest clearly rises with rescue breaths, the victim starts breathing, or the ambulance arrives

This booklet is not a substitute for materials used in American Red Cross courses in which First Aid or CPR certification is given.

CHOKING —
UNCONSCIOUS ADULT

1

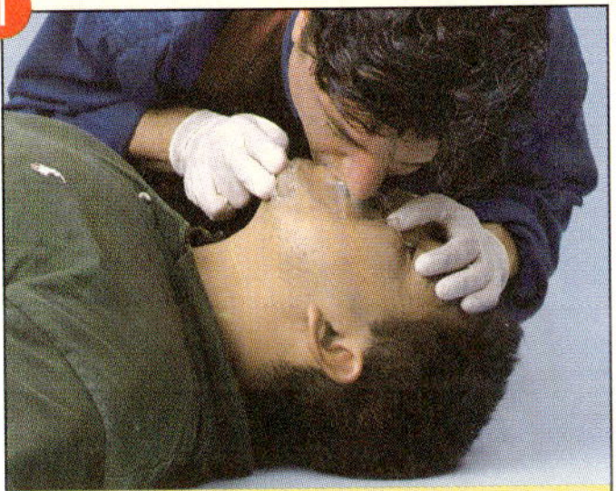

- Attempt to give breaths. If you can't get air in, reposition airway and reattempt breaths

2

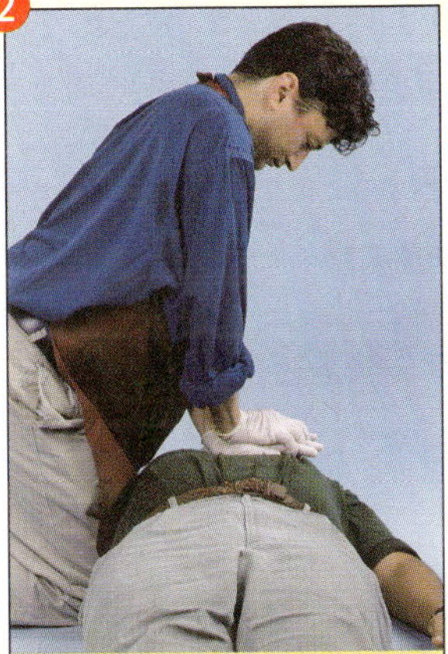

- Find hand position
- Position shoulders over hands
- Compress chest 15 times

3

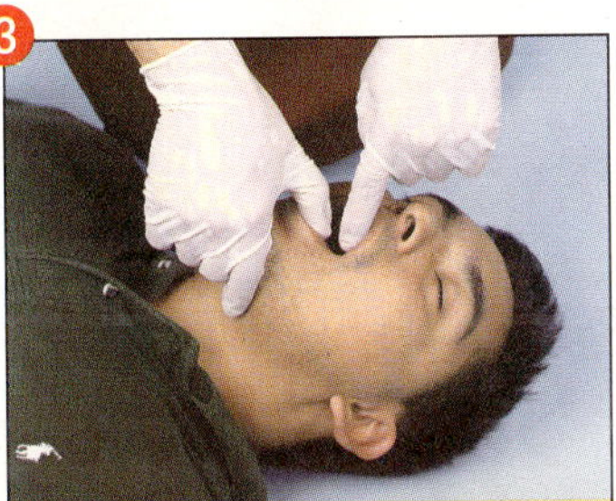

- Look into the mouth. Remove object if seen
- Repeat steps beginning with 2 rescue breaths until you can breathe into victim, making the chest clearly rise

CHOKING —
UNCONSCIOUS CHILD

The airway can be blocked by the tongue falling back in the throat or by a small object, such as food or toys.

SIGNAL

- Unable to make chest clearly rise when attempting rescue breaths

CARE

- Send someone to CALL 9-1-1 or the local emergency number. If alone, provide 1 minute of care before calling
- Tilt head back, lift chin, and pinch nose shut
- Give 2 slow rescue breaths. Breathe in until chest clearly rises
- If chest does not rise while giving breaths, REPOSITION airway and reattempt breaths

If breaths still do not go in:

- Place the heel of one hand in center of chest over breastbone
- Position shoulder over hand
- Compress chest 5 times in about 3 seconds
- Lift lower jaw and tongue and look for object in mouth. If object is visible, remove it with your little finger
- Tilt head back, lift chin, and pinch nose shut, and give 1 slow rescue breath

If breaths still do not go in:

- Continue sets of 5 compressions, followed by look for an object/ removal and 1 rescue breath until chest clearly rises with rescue breaths, the child starts breathing, or the ambulance arrives

CHOKING —
UNCONSCIOUS CHILD

1

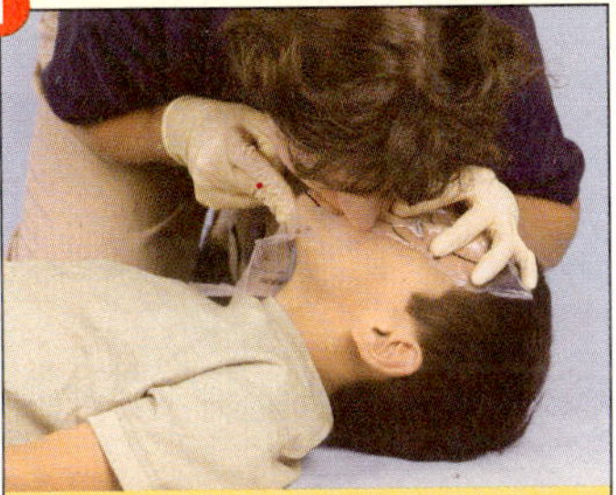

- Attempt to give breaths. If you can't get air in, reposition airway and reattempt breaths

2

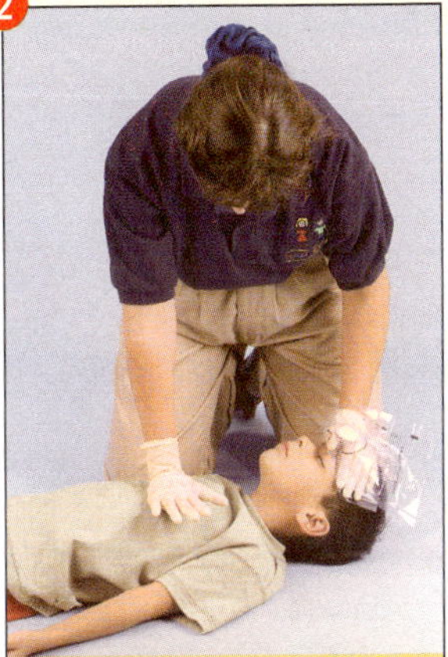

- Position shoulder over hand
- Compress chest 5 times

3

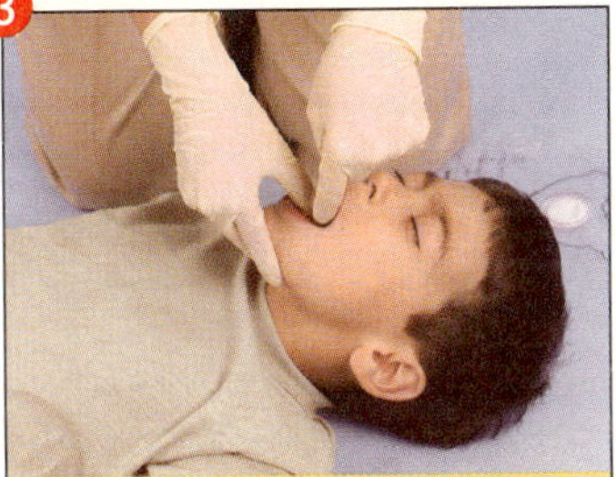

- Look in the mouth. Remove object if seen
- Repeat steps beginning with 1 rescue breath until you can breathe into victim, making the chest clearly rise

CHOKING —
CONSCIOUS INFANT

Choking is a major cause of death and injury in infants. Infants can easily choke on toys or food, such as nuts, grapes, and popcorn.

SIGNALS

- Coughing forcefully for several minutes without result
- Cannot cry, cough, or breathe
- Coughing weakly or making high-pitched sounds

CARE

- CHECK the scene and the infant
- Send someone to CALL 9-1-1 or the local emergency number. If alone, provide 1 minute of care before calling
- With infant facedown on forearm, give 5 back blows with the heel of the hand between the shoulder blades. Support the infant's head and neck
- Position infant face up on your forearm
- Give 5 thrusts in the center of the breastbone with your middle and index fingers

Repeat back blows and chest thrusts until object is coughed up and infant begins to breathe on own or becomes unconscious.

If infant becomes unconscious, look for an object in the mouth. If object is seen, remove it with your little finger. Continue with care for Choking — Unconscious Infant (pp. 38-39)

CHOKING —
CONSCIOUS INFANT

1

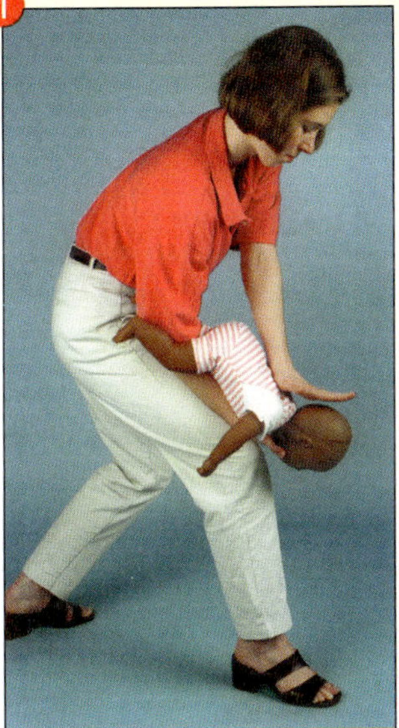

- Give 5 back blows

2

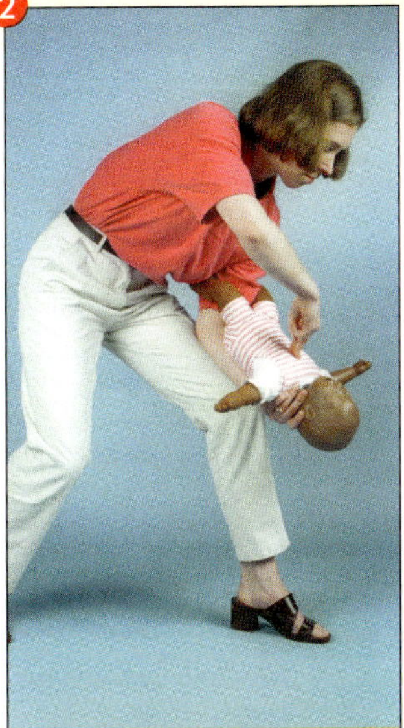

- Give 5 chest thrusts
- Repeat back blows and chest thrusts until object is coughed up and infant begins to breathe on own or becomes unconscious

CHOKING —
UNCONSCIOUS INFANT

The airway can be blocked by the tongue falling back in the throat or by a small object, such as food or toys.

SIGNAL

- Unable to make the chest clearly rise when attempting rescue breaths

CARE

- Send someone to CALL 9-1-1 or the local emergency number. If alone, provide 1 minute of care before calling
- Cover infant's mouth and nose with your mouth and give 2 slow rescue breaths until chest clearly rises
- If chest does not rise while giving breaths, REPOSITION the airway and reattempt breaths

If breaths still do not go in:

- Place two fingers in center of chest over breastbone
- Position hand over fingers
- Compress chest 5 times in slightly less than 3 seconds
- Lift lower jaw and tongue and look for object in mouth. If object is visible, remove it with your little finger
- Tilt head back, cover the mouth and nose, and give 1 slow rescue breath

If breaths still do not go in:

- Continue sets of 5 compressions, followed by look for an object/removal and 1 rescue breath until chest clearly rises with rescue breaths, infant starts breathing, or the ambulance arrives

CHOKING —
UNCONSCIOUS INFANT

1

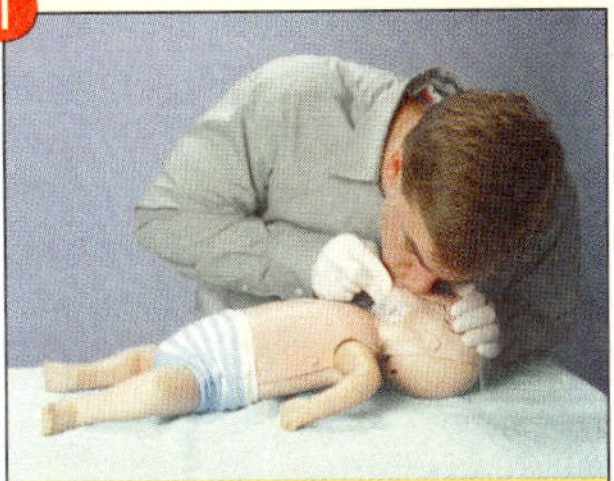

- Attempt to give breaths. If you can't get air in, reposition airway and reattempt breaths

2

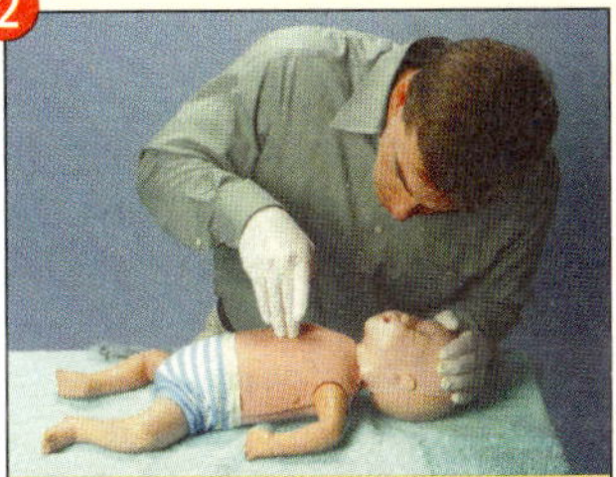

- Position hand over fingers
- Compress chest 5 times

3

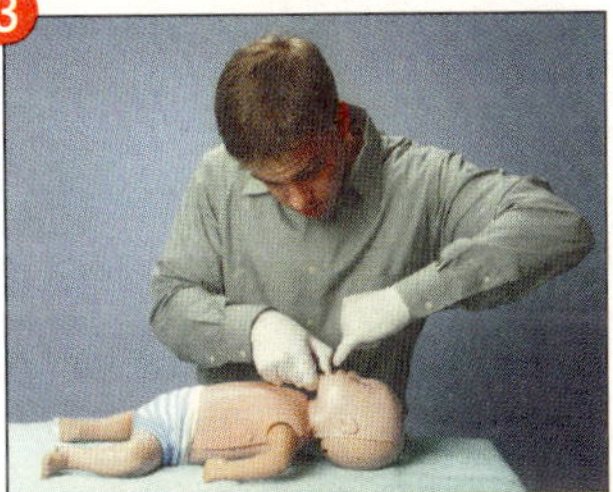

- Look into the mouth. Remove object if seen
- Repeat steps beginning with 1 rescue breath until you can breathe into the infant, making the chest clearly rise

COLD-RELATED ILLNESS

Hypothermia and frostbite are two types of cold-related emergencies. BOTH conditions can quickly become life- or limb-threatening. *Hypothermia* is the cooling of the body caused by the failure of the body's warming system. *Frostbite* is the freezing of body parts.

HYPOTHERMIA

SIGNALS

- Shivering, numbness, glassy stare
- Apathy, weakness, impaired judgement
- Loss of consciousness

CARE

- CHECK the scene and the person
- Send someone to CALL 9-1-1 or the local emergency number
- GENTLY move person to a warm place
- Give rescue breathing (see Breathing Emergencies — p. 12) or CPR (see Cardiac Emergencies — pp. 25-29) if needed
- Remove any wet clothing and dry the person
- Warm person SLOWLY by wrapping in blankets or by putting dry clothing on person. Hot water bottles and chemical hot packs may be used when first wrapped in a towel or blanket before applying
- DO NOT WARM PERSON TOO QUICKLY, such as immersing him or her in warm water. Rapid warming can cause dangerous heart rhythms

This booklet is not a substitute for materials used in American Red Cross courses in which First Aid or CPR certification is given.

I'm ready to train with the American Red Cross!

To order additional copies of *First Aid Fast*, **contact your local American Red Cross chapter or call**

1-800-667-2968.

American Red Cross

Together, we can save a life

YES! Please send me more information on American Red Cross courses and products in:

- ❑ *First aid*
- ❑ *CPR/Automated External Defibrillation (AED)*
- ❑ *Swimming and water safety*
- ❑ *Lifeguarding*
- ❑ *Nurse assistant training*
- ❑ *Babysitter's training*
- ❑ *HIV/AIDS education*
- ❑ *Preventing disease transmission*
- ❑ *Oxygen administration*
- ❑ *Professional level first aid and CPR*

Name:____

Organization:___________________________________

Address:______________________________________

City:____

State:____

Zip:____

Daytime phone:__________________________________

What is the best time to reach you?__________________

E-mail address:_________________________________

American Red Cross

Together, we can save a life

American Red Cross

Together, we can save a life

NO POSTAGE
NECESSARY
IF MAILED
IN THE
UNITED STATES

BUSINESS REPLY MAIL

FIRST-CLASS MAIL   PERMIT NO. 3   SAN BRUNO, CA

POSTAGE WILL BE PAID BY ADDRESSEE

AMERICAN RED CROSS CUSTOMER RELATIONS
KRAMES/STAYWELL
1100 GRUNDY LANE
SAN BRUNO CA 94066-9821

COLD-RELATED ILLNESS

FROSTBITE

SIGNALS

- Lack of feeling in the affected area
- Skin appears waxy, is cold to the touch, or is discolored (flushed, white, gray, yellow, or blue)

CARE

- CHECK the scene and the person
- Send someone to CALL 9-1-1 or the local emergency number
- Attempt to remove jewelry or restrictive clothing
- Handle the area gently; never rub the affected area
- Warm gently by soaking affected area in warm water (100 degrees Fahrenheit to 105 degrees Fahrenheit) until it appears red and feels warm
- Loosely bandage area with dry, sterile dressing
- If the victim's fingers or toes are frostbitten, place dry, sterile gauze between them to keep them separated
- Avoid breaking any blisters

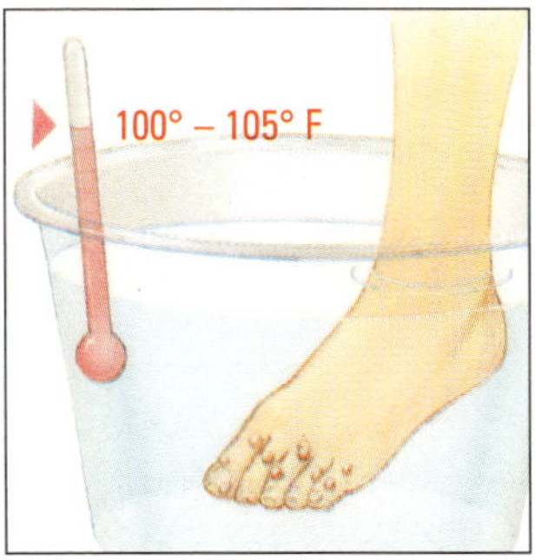

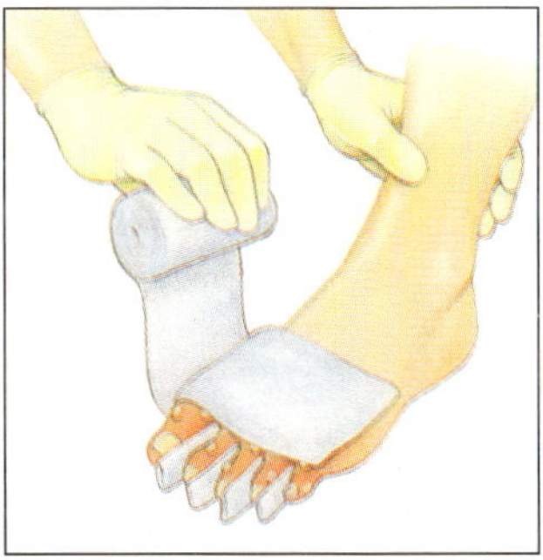

HEAT-RELATED ILLNESS

Heat cramps and heat-related illness are progressive conditions caused by overexposure to heat. If recognized in the early stages, heat-related illness can usually be reversed. If not, it may progress to a life-threatening condition.

HEAT CRAMPS

SIGNAL

- Painful muscle spasms, usually in the legs and abdomen

CARE

- Have person rest in a cool place
- Give cool water to drink
- Lightly stretch and gently massage the muscle
- DO NOT GIVE SALT TABLETS
- Watch for signals of heat illness

This booklet is not a substitute for materials used in American Red Cross courses in which First Aid or CPR certification is given.

HEAT-RELATED ILLNESS

HEAT ILLNESS

SIGNALS

Early Stages:

- Cool, moist, pale, or flushed skin
- Headache, nausea, dizziness
- Weakness, exhaustion
- Heavy sweating

Late Stages:

- Red, hot, dry skin
- Changes in level of consciousness
- Vomiting

CARE

- Move person to a cool place
- Loosen tight or remove perspiration-soaked clothing
- Apply cool, wet cloths to the skin or mist with cool water and fan the person
- If conscious, give cool water to drink

If person refuses water, vomits, or loses consciousness:

- Send someone to CALL 9-1-1 or the local emergency number and place person on his or her side
- Continue to cool by placing ice or cold packs on person's wrists, ankles, groin, and neck and in armpits
- If the victim becomes unconscious, give rescue breathing (see Breathing Emergencies — p. 12) or CPR (see Cardiac Emergencies — pp. 25-29) if needed

INJURIES TO —
MUSCLES, BONES, AND JOINTS

Only a trained medical professional can tell the difference between a sprain, strain, fracture, or dislocation. You do not need to know what kind of injury it is to give the correct first aid.

SIGNALS

- Pain
- Bruising and swelling

CARE

- CHECK the scene and the person
- Rest the injured part
- Apply ice or a cold pack to control swelling and reduce pain. Place a towel or cloth between the source of cold and the skin
- Avoid any movement or activity that causes pain

If you suspect a serious injury:

- Immobilize the injured part to keep it from moving
- Send someone to CALL 9-1-1 or the local emergency number

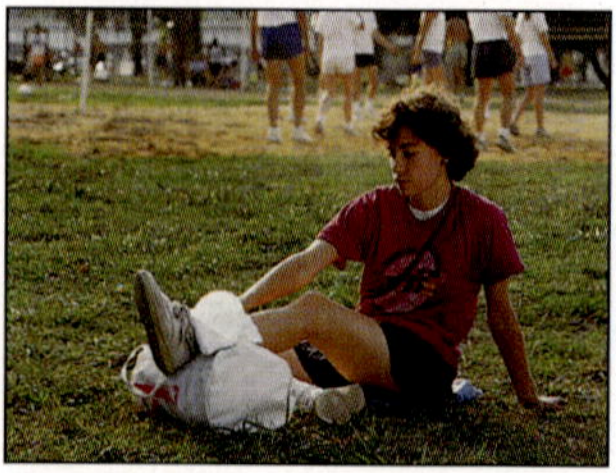

This booklet is not a substitute for materials used in American Red Cross courses in which First Aid or CPR certification is given.

INJURIES TO —
MUSCLES, BONES, AND JOINTS

WHEN TO CALL 9-1-1 OR THE LOCAL EMERGENCY NUMBER

- Feels or sounds like bones are rubbing together
- "Snap" or "pop" heard or felt at time of injury
- An open wound on or around the injury site; bone ends may or may not be visible
- Inability to move or use the affected part normally
- Injured area is cold and numb
- Injury involves the head, neck, or back
- Person has trouble breathing
- Cause of the injury suggests that the injury may be severe

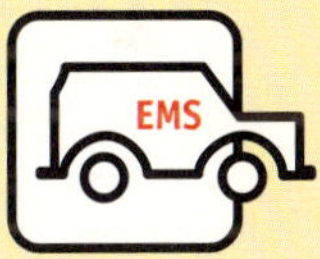

INJURIES TO —
MUSCLES, BONES, AND JOINTS

SPLINTING

Splinting is a method to keep an injured body part from moving. It can also help to reduce pain, making the injured person more comfortable.

- Splint only if the person must be moved or transported and if you can do so without causing more pain and discomfort to the person
- Splint an injury in the position you find it
- Splint the joints above and below an injured bone
- Splint the bones above and below an injured joint
- Check for feeling, warmth and color of the skin below the site of injury both before and after splinting

INJURIES TO —
MUSCLES, BONES, AND JOINTS

SPLINTING METHODS

There are a variety of ways to splint an injured body part. When choosing a method, consider what materials you have available and what will best keep the injured part from moving. Often, simply supporting the injured part in the position you find it — such as placing a small pillow or folded blanket under an injured leg against the ground — is the best method of all.

Anatomic splint

A part of the body is used as a splint (an injured leg can be splinted to an uninjured leg)

Soft splint

Made with soft materials such as folded blankets, towels, or pillows

Sling

A triangular bandage tied to support an injured arm, wrist, or hand

Rigid splint

Made with boards, folded magazines, newspaper, or metal strips

INJURIES TO —
MUSCLES, BONES, AND JOINTS

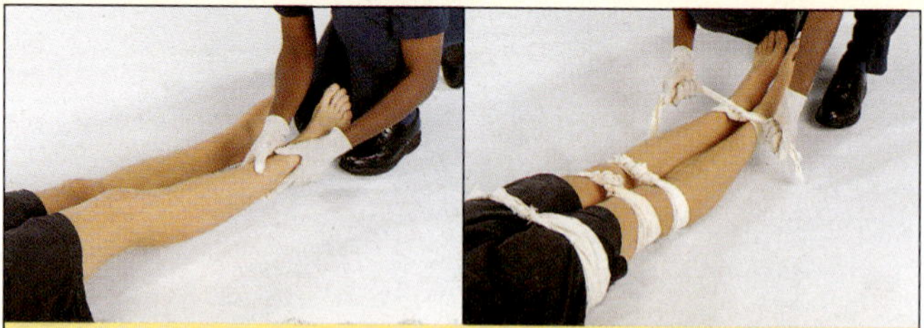

Anatomic splint

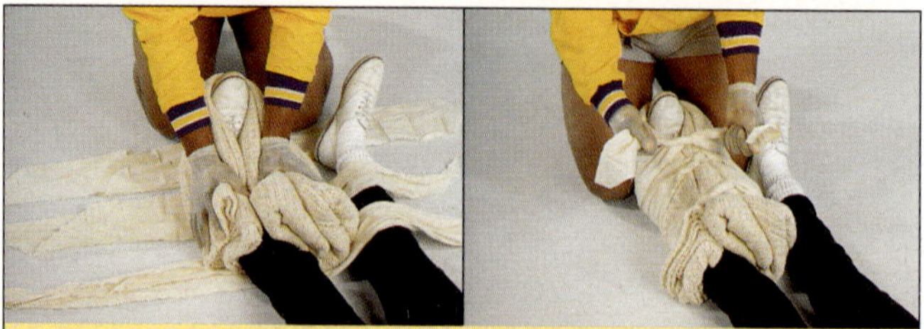

Soft splint

This booklet is not a substitute for materials used in American Red Cross courses in which First Aid or CPR certification is given.

INJURIES TO —
MUSCLES, BONES, AND JOINTS

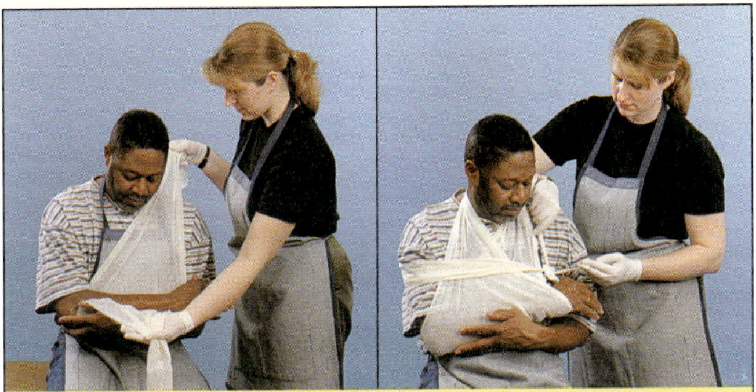

Sling

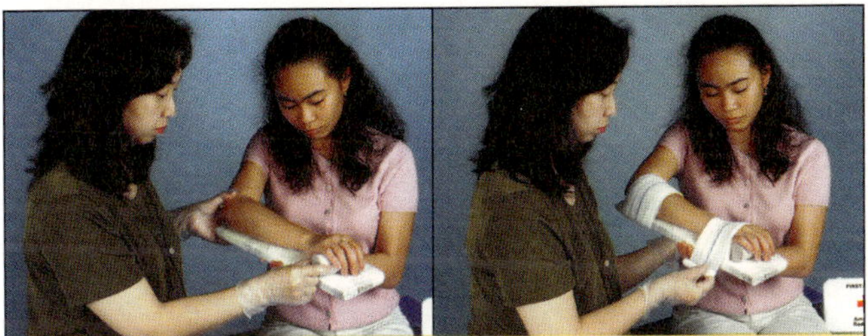

Rigid splint

INJURIES TO —

HEAD, NECK, AND BACK

Although injuries to the head, neck, and back account for only a small percentage of all injuries, they cause more than half of all injury-related deaths. Signals of a head, neck, or back injury may be sometimes slow to develop and are not always noticeable at first.

ALWAYS SUSPECT A HEAD, NECK, OR BACK INJURY IN THESE SITUATIONS

- A fall from a height greater than the person's height
- Any diving mishap
- A person found unconscious for unknown reasons
- Any injury involving severe blunt force to the head or trunk, such as from a motor vehicle
- Any injury that penetrates the head or trunk, such as a gunshot wound
- A motor vehicle crash involving a driver or passengers not wearing safety belts
- Any person thrown from a motor vehicle
- Any injury in which a person's helmet is broken, including a motorcycle, football, or industrial helmet
- Any incident involving a lightning strike

INJURIES TO —
HEAD, NECK, AND BACK

SIGNALS

- Changes in consciousness, loss of balance, seizures
- Severe pain or pressure in the head, neck, or back
- Tingling or loss of sensation in the hands, fingers, feet, or toes
- Partial or complete loss of movement of any body part
- Unusual bumps or depressions on the head or over the spine
- Blood or other fluids draining from the ears or nose
- Heavy external bleeding from the head, neck, or back
- Impaired breathing or vision as a result of injury
- Nausea, vomiting, or persistent headache
- Bruising of the head, especially around the eyes and behind the ears

INJURIES TO —
HEAD, NECK, AND BACK

CARE

- CHECK the scene and the person
- Send someone to CALL 9-1-1 or the local emergency number
- Keep the person's head, neck, and back from moving
- CHECK consciousness and breathing. If the person is not breathing, use the jaw-thrust maneuver to open airway
- Place one hand on each side of the victim's head with your thumbs on the victim's cheeks and your fingers under the back of the lower jaw, next to the ears
- Grab the back of the lower jaw, next to the ears, and lift with both hands
- Maintain a clear, open airway. Do not move the victim unnecessarily. If the person is not breathing, place your cheek tightly against the victim's nose
- Give two slow breaths
- CHECK for movement (coughing or response to breaths). Give rescue breathing (see Breathing Emergencies — p. 12) or CPR (see Cardiac Emergencies — pp. 25-29) if needed
- Control bleeding
- Keep victim from getting chilled or overheated
- DO NOT MOVE PERSON UNLESS ABSOLUTELY NECESSARY. If the person must be moved, do it carefully without twisting or bending the body. If alone, use the person's clothes to drag the person to safety while supporting the head and neck in the best way possible

INJURIES TO —
HEAD, NECK, AND BACK

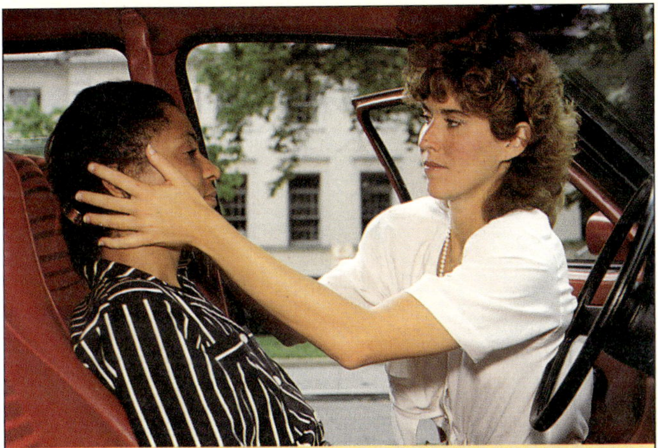

- If you suspect an injury to the head, neck, or back, support the person's head in line with the body

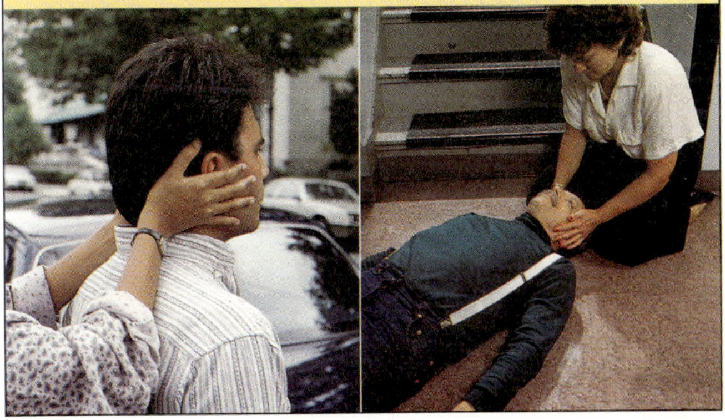

POISONING

A poison is a substance that causes injury or illness if it gets into the body. There are four ways a poison can enter the body — by swallowing it, breathing it, touching it, or having it injected. Combinations of certain substances, such as drugs and alcohol, can be poisonous, although if taken by themselves they might not cause harm. Not everyone reacts to poisons in the same way. A substance that is harmful to one may not always be harmful to another.

SIGNALS

- Trouble breathing
- Nausea, vomiting, diarrhea
- Chest or abdominal pain
- Sweating, changes in consciousness, seizures
- Burns around the lips, tongue, or on the skin
- Open or spilled containers; open medicine cabinet
- Overturned or damaged plant
- Unusual odors, flames, smoke

POISONING

POISON CONTROL CENTERS

Many poisonings can be cared for without the help of ambulance personnel. The people who staff Poison Control Centers (PCCs) have access to information on most poisonous substances and can tell you what care to give to counteract the poison.

Keep your PCC telephone number posted by the telephone. Also record it on the last page of this guide. You may find the number of your PCC in the inside front cover of the phone book.

POISONING

CARE

- CHECK the scene to make sure it is safe to approach and gather clues about what happened
- If necessary, move the person to safety, away from the source of the poison
- CHECK the victim's level of consciousness, breathing, and movement (coughing or response to rescue breaths). CARE for any life-threatening conditions
- Send someone to CALL 9-1-1 or the local emergency number or Poison Control Center as necessary
- Look for any containers
- If you suspect someone has swallowed a poison, try to find out what type of poison it was, how much was taken, and when it was taken
- NEVER GIVE ANYTHING TO EAT OR DRINK UNLESS DIRECTED TO DO SO BY THE POISON CONTROL CENTER OR HEALTH CARE PROVIDER
- If the person vomits, position on side. Save a sample of the vomit if poison is not known so that it can be identified at the hospital

POISONING —
ALLERGIC REACTIONS

Allergic reactions to certain foods and bee stings can cause severe swelling of the face and air passages, restricting breathing.

SIGNALS

- Trouble breathing
- Feeling of tightness in the chest and throat
- Swelling of the face, neck, and tongue
- Rash, hives, dizziness, or confusion

CARE

- CHECK the scene to make sure it is safe
- CHECK the person carefully for swelling and breathing problems
- If the person has trouble breathing, send someone to CALL the Poison Control Center, 9-1-1 or the local emergency number
- People who know they are allergic may carry a special kit

CARING FOR BITES AND STINGS

INSECT BITES/STINGS

SIGNALS

- Stinger may be present
- Pain
- Swelling
- Possible allergic reactions

CARE

- Remove stinger — scrape it away or use tweezers
- Wash wound
- Cover
- Apply a cold pack
- Watch for signals of allergic reaction

SPIDER BITES/SCORPION STINGS

SIGNALS

- Bite mark
- Swelling
- Pain
- Nausea and vomiting
- Trouble breathing or swallowing

CARE

- Wash wound
- Apply a cold pack
- Get medical care to receive antivenin
- Call 9-1-1 or the local emergency number, if necessary

This booklet is not a substitute for materials used in American Red Cross courses in which First Aid or CPR certification is given.

CARING FOR BITES AND STINGS

MARINE LIFE STINGS

SIGNALS

- Possible marks
- Pain
- Swelling
- Possible allergic reaction

CARE

- If jellyfish — soak area in vinegar
- If sting ray — soak area in nonscalding hot water until pain goes away. Clean and bandage wound
- Call 9-1-1 or the local emergency number, if necessary

SNAKE BITES

SIGNALS

- Bite mark
- Pain

CARE

- Wash wound
- Keep bitten part still, and lower than the heart
- Call 9-1-1 or the local emergency number

ANIMAL BITES

SIGNALS

- Bite mark
- Pain

CARE

- If bleeding is minor — wash wound
- Control bleeding
- Apply antibiotic ointment
- Cover
- Get medical attention if wound bleeds severely or if you suspect animal has rabies
- Call 9-1-1 or the local emergency number or contact animal control personnel

POISONING —
SPECIAL SITUATIONS

DRY AND WET CHEMICALS

- CHECK the scene to make sure it is safe
- Send someone to CALL 9-1-1 or the local emergency number, if necessary
- For a wet chemical, flush affected areas with large amounts of cool running water until ambulance arrives. Always flush away from the body. Brush dry chemicals off the skin with a gloved hand
- Remove clothing and jewelry that may trap chemical against the skin or on which chemicals may have spilled

POISONOUS PLANTS

- Immediately wash the affected area thoroughly with soap and water
- If a rash or open sores develop, apply paste of baking soda and water several times a day to reduce discomfort
- Lotions, such as Caladryl™, may help soothe the area
- If condition gets worse or affects large areas of the body or face, see a doctor

POISONING —

TICK BITES AND LYME DISEASE

Not all ticks carry Lyme disease. It is spread mainly by a small type of tick found around wooded and grassy areas. Proper clothing and frequent checks for ticks can prevent tick bites. Signals of Lyme disease might develop slowly and might not occur at the same time as a rash. You can have Lyme disease without developing a rash.

SIGNALS

- Rash starts as a small red area at the site of the bite; may appear a few days or a few weeks after the bite
- Fair skin: the center may be lighter in color and the outer edges are red and raised (bull's eye appearance)
- Dark skin: the area may look black and blue
- Fever, headache, weakness
- Flu-like joint and muscle pain

CARE

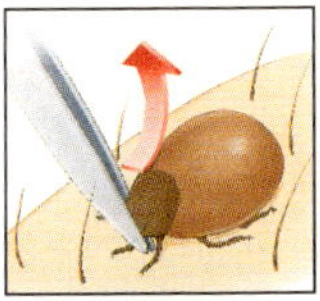

- Grasp tick with fine-tipped tweezers close to skin and pull slowly. Use plastic wrap, paper, or leaf if you do not have tweezers
- DO NOT try to burn tick off. DO NOT apply petroleum jelly or nail polish to tick
- If you cannot remove tick, or if its mouthparts remain imbedded, get medical care
- Wash bite area with soap and water. Apply antibiotic ointment
- If rash or flu-like signals appear, see your health care provider immediately

REACHING AND MOVING VICTIMS

Moving a person can make some injuries worse. You should move a person only if there is immediate danger or the person has to be moved to give proper care. Even if you are in a remote area, such as when camping, it is often easier to bring professional medical help to the injured or ill person than the person to the help. Once you decide to move someone, you must determine how to move them. Always consider your safety and the safety of the person.

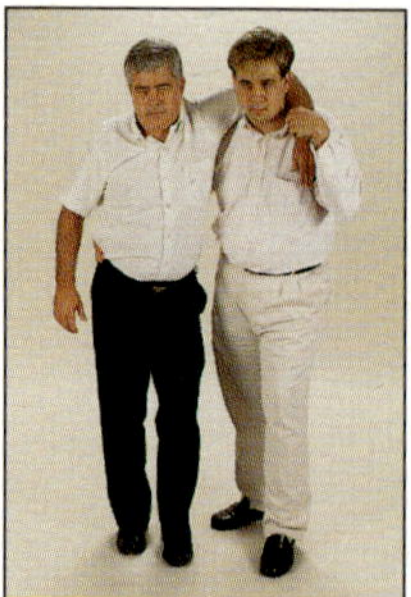

Walking assist

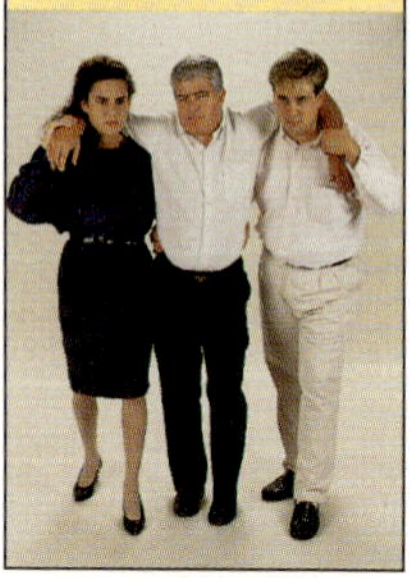

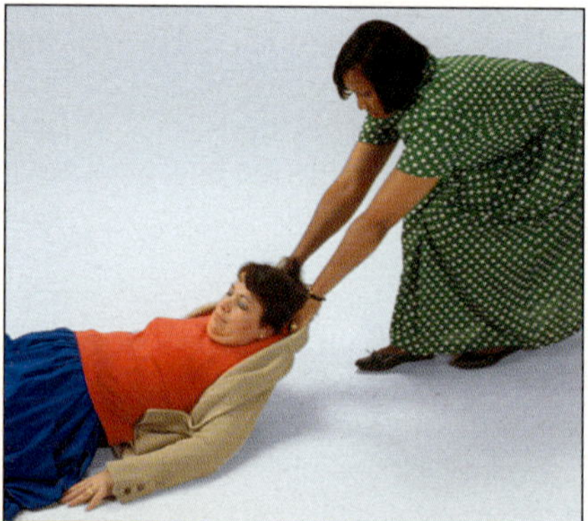

Clothes drag

This booklet is not a substitute for materials used in American Red Cross courses in which First Aid or CPR certification is given.

REACHING AND MOVING VICTIMS

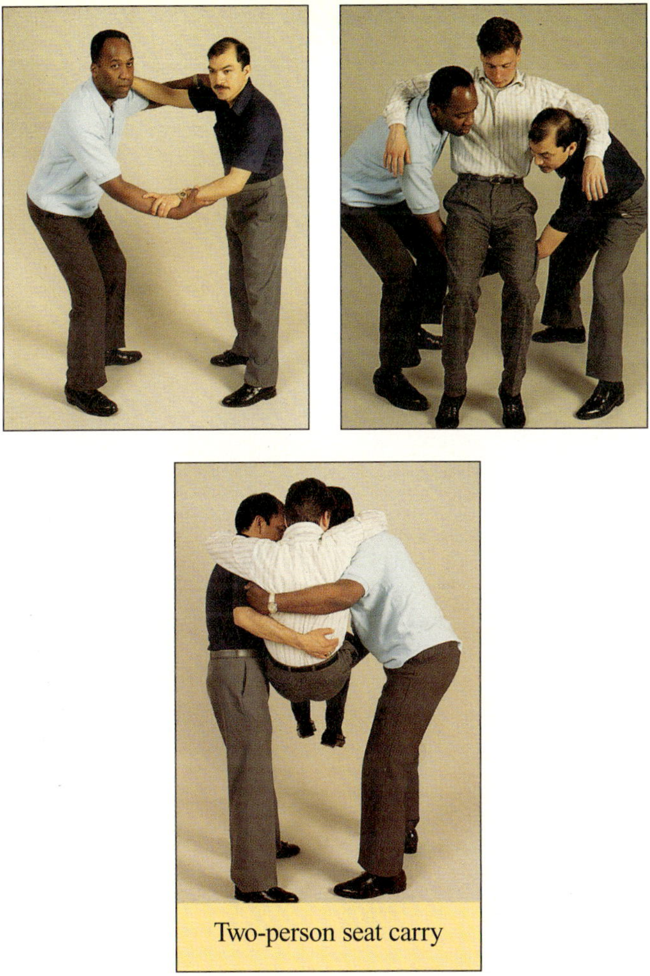

Two-person seat carry

REACHING AND MOVING VICTIMS —

WATER RESCUES

Emergencies can happen to anyone in or around the water, regardless of how good a swimmer the person is or the nature of the activity. Drownings often occur to persons who never intended to get wet. Drownings can also happen in the home in as little water as a bucket or tubful. Being able to recognize a person who is having trouble in the water may help save the person's life. Stay alert and know the signals that indicate an emergency — the victim may not be able to call for help!

SIGNALS

- Struggling movements; little or no forward progress
- Person may or may not be able to call or signal for help
- Person struggles to breathe

CARE

- CHECK the scene for safety
- Send someone to CALL 9-1-1 or the local emergency number
- Attempt to rescue by reaching or throwing an object that floats to the person. DO NOT ATTEMPT A SWIMMING RESCUE UNLESS YOU HAVE PROPER EQUIPMENT AND ARE TRAINED TO DO SO

Once the person is out of the water:

- CHECK the person. Care for any conditions you find

REACHING AND MOVING VICTIMS —

WATER RESCUES

The safest methods are reaching, throwing, and wading assists. In most cases, at least one of these methods will succeed.

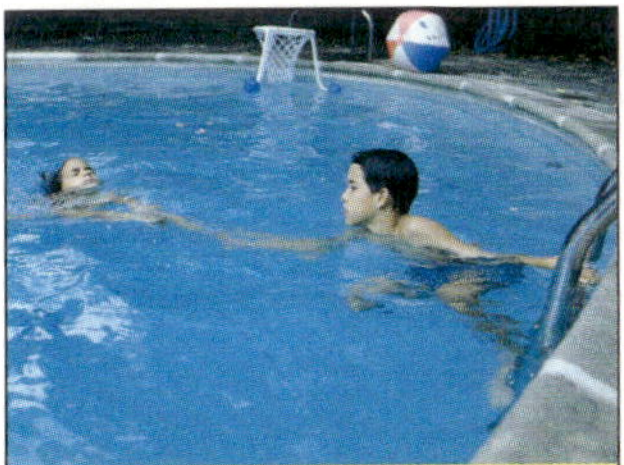

Reaching assists

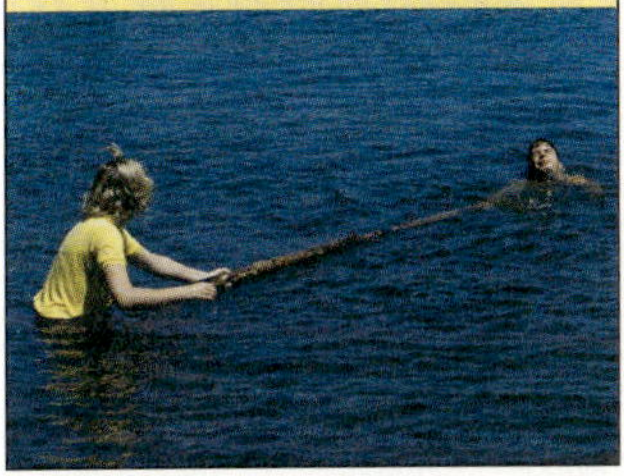

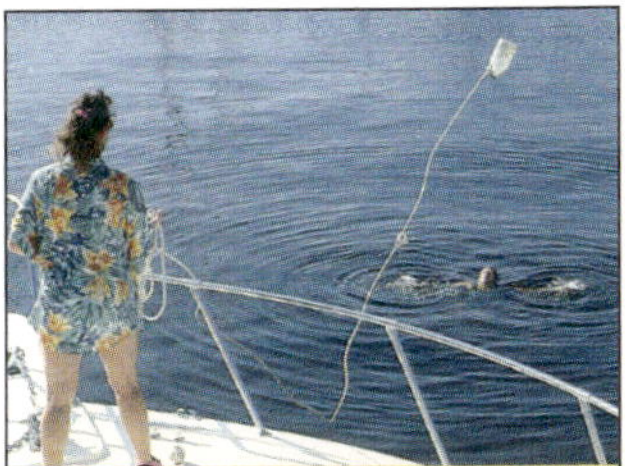

Throwing assist

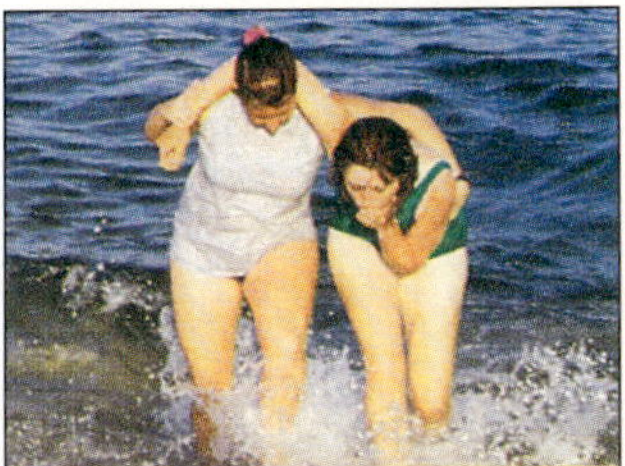

Wading assist

SUDDEN ILLNESS

Many different types of sudden illnesses often have similar signals. Usually you will not know the exact cause of the illness, but this should not keep you from providing care. Care for the signals you find.

SIGNALS

- Feeling light-headed, dizzy, confused, or weak
- Changes in skin color (pale or flushed skin), sweating
- Nausea, vomiting, or diarrhea

Some illnesses may also include:

- Seizure or changes in consciousness
- Paralysis (inability to move), slurred speech, or difficulty seeing
- Severe headache, trouble breathing, persistent pressure, or pain

CARE

- Send someone to CALL 9-1-1 or the local emergency number, if necessary
- CARE for any life-threatening conditions first
- Help person rest comfortably
- Keep person from getting chilled or overheated
- Reassure the person
- Watch for changes in consciousness, breathing, and movement (coughing or response to rescue breaths)
- Do not give anything to eat or drink unless person is fully conscious

This booklet is not a substitute for materials used in American Red Cross courses in which First Aid or CPR certification is given.

SUDDEN ILLNESS

WHEN TO CALL 9-1-1 OR THE LOCAL EMERGENCY NUMBER

- Person is unconscious, unusually confused, or seems to be losing consciousness
- Person has trouble breathing or is breathing in a strange way
- Person has persistent chest pain or pressure
- Person has pressure or pain in the abdomen that does not go away
- Person is vomiting or passing blood
- Person has seizures, severe headache, or slurred speech
- Person appears to have been poisoned
- Person has injuries to the head, neck, or back

— OR —

- You can't sort the problem out quickly and easily or you have doubts about the severity of the illness

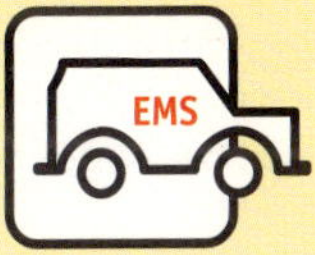

SUDDEN ILLNESS —
SPECIAL SITUATIONS

SEIZURES

If you know the person has epilepsy, it is usually not necessary to call 9-1-1 or the local emergency number unless: the seizure lasts longer than 5 minutes or is repeated; the person does not regain consciousness; or the person is pregnant, known to be a diabetic, is injured, or shows other life-threatening conditions.

CARE

- Send someone to CALL 9-1-1 or the local emergency number, if necessary
- Remove nearby objects that might cause injury
- Protect the person's head by placing a folded towel or clothing beneath it
- Do not hold or restrain person
- Do not place anything between the person's teeth
- Place the person on the side to drain fluids from mouth
- When seizure is over, CHECK for breathing and injuries
- Comfort person. Stay until person is fully conscious

STROKE

A stroke is caused by a lack of oxygen to the brain when a blood vessel bursts or becomes narrowed by a clot.

CARE

- Send someone to CALL 9-1-1 or the local emergency number
- CARE for the specific conditions you find
- If person is drooling or having difficulty swallowing, place person on his or her side to keep airway clear

SUDDEN ILLNESS —
SPECIAL SITUATIONS

FAINTING

Fainting is a temporary loss of consciousness. It may indicate a more serious condition.

CARE

- Send someone to CALL 9-1-1 or the local emergency number, if necessary
- Elevate legs 8 to 12 inches if injury is not suspected
- Loosen any tight clothing
- Check breathing and movement (coughing or response to rescue breaths)
- Do not give anything to eat or drink

DIABETIC EMERGENCY

Diabetes is a condition where the body is unable to balance insulin and sugar in the body. Diabetics sometimes become ill because there is too much or too little sugar in their blood. In either case, giving sugar will not cause additional harm.

CARE

- If person is conscious and a known diabetic, give sugar (fruit juices, nondiet drinks, table sugar)
- If person is not feeling better in about 5 minutes, CALL 9-1-1 or the local emergency number
- If person is unconscious, DO NOT GIVE ANYTHING TO EAT OR DRINK. Send someone to CALL 9-1-1 or the local emergency number. Give care for the conditions you find

WOUNDS

A wound is an injury to the skin and soft tissues beneath it. Damage to blood vessels causes bleeding. When caring for wounds, it is important to take precautions to protect yourself against the transmission of disease.

Follow these simple procedures:

- When possible, ask the injured person to help you
- Wear disposable gloves or place a barrier between you and the person's blood
- Wash hands with soap and water immediately before and after providing care

SIGNALS

- Cuts, scrapes, punctures, or other breaks in the skin
- Bleeding, bruising; area may swell

WOUNDS

WHEN TO CALL 9-1-1 OR THE LOCAL EMERGENCY NUMBER

- Bleeding that cannot be stopped
- Wounds that show muscle or bone, involve joints, are deep, or involve hands or feet
- Large wounds
- Large or deeply imbedded objects in the wound
- Human or animal bites
- Any wound that would leave an obvious scar, such as on the face
- Skin or body parts that have been partially or completely torn away

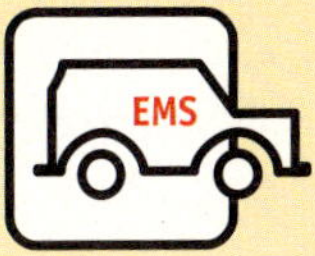

WOUNDS

CARE

- CHECK the scene for safety
- Send someone to CALL 9-1-1 or the local emergency number
- Cover the wound with a sterile gauze pad and press firmly against the wound (use your bare hand to apply pressure only as a last resort)
- If dressing becomes soaked with blood, do not remove it. Apply additional dressing on top
- ELEVATE the injured area above the level of the heart if you do not suspect broken bones or head, neck, or back injury
- Cover gauze dressings with a roller bandage to maintain pressure

If bleeding doesn't stop:

- Apply additional dressings and bandage
- Squeeze the nearby artery against the bone underneath

  Arm: Inside of the upper arm, between the shoulder and elbow

  Leg: Crease at the front of the hip, in the groin

This booklet is not a substitute for materials used in American Red Cross courses in which First Aid or CPR certification is given.

WOUNDS —
CONTROLLING BLEEDING

1

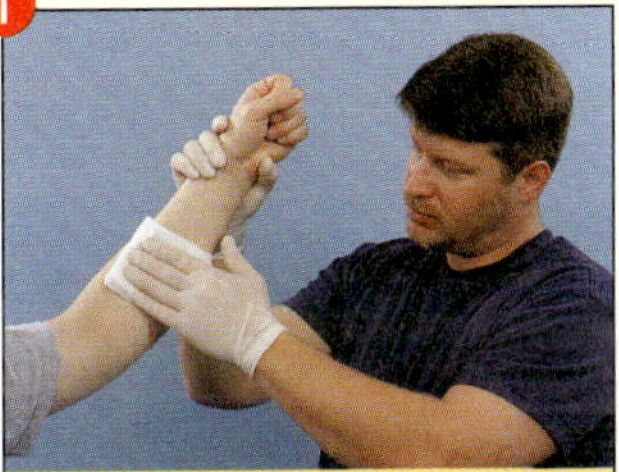

- Apply direct pressure and elevation

2

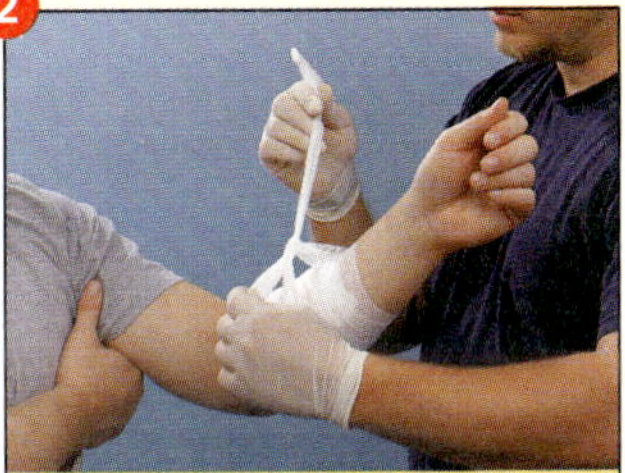

- Apply a bandage

3

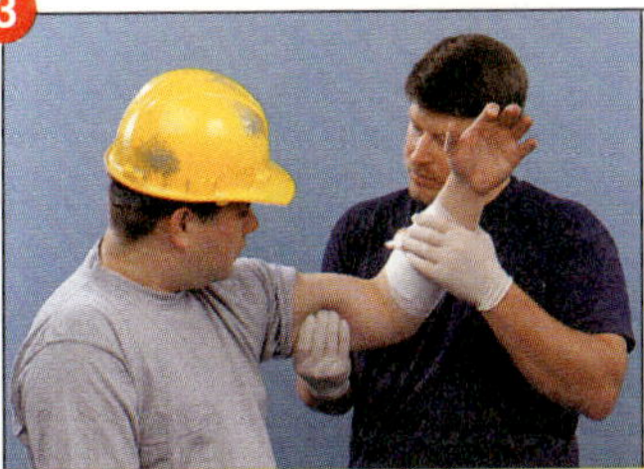

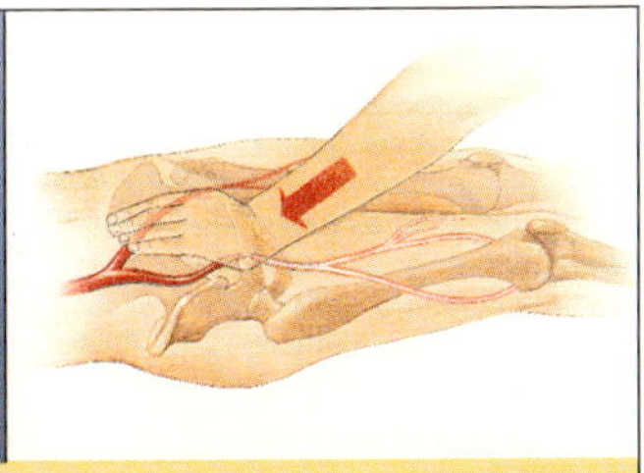

ARM **If bleeding doesn't stop:** LEG

- Apply pressure to a nearby artery

WOUNDS —
SPECIAL SITUATIONS

BRUISES

- Apply ice or a cold pack to help control pain and swelling. Place a cloth between source of cold and skin to prevent injury
- Elevate injured part to reduce swelling

SEVERED BODY PARTS

- Wrap severed body part in sterile gauze or clean cloth
- Place severed part in a plastic bag
- Put the plastic bag on ice and take to hospital with person

IMBEDDED OBJECT

- Send someone to CALL 9-1-1 or the local emergency number
- DO NOT REMOVE OBJECT
- Bandage bulky dressings around the object to support object in place
- Bandage the dressing in place

NOSEBLEED

- Have person lean slightly forward
- Pinch the nose shut for about 10 minutes
- Apply an ice pack to the bridge of the nose

If bleeding doesn't stop:

- Apply pressure on upper lip just beneath nose

This booklet is not a substitute for materials used in American Red Cross courses in which First Aid or CPR certification is given.

WOUNDS —
SPECIAL SITUATIONS

CHEST

- Send someone to CALL 9-1-1 or the local emergency number
- Cover the wound with a sterile dressing or clean cloth and bandage in place
- If bubbles are forming around wound, cover with plastic or material that does not allow air to pass through. Tape dressing in place, leaving one corner open to allow air to escape when person exhales

MOUTH AND CHEEK

If no serious head, neck, or back injury is suspected:

- Have person lean slightly forward or place on his or her side
- For inside the cheek: Place folded sterile dressings inside the mouth against wound
- For outside the cheek: Apply direct pressure using a sterile dressing
- For tongue or lips: Apply direct pressure using a sterile dressing. Apply cold to reduce swelling and ease pain

WOUNDS —
SPECIAL SITUATIONS

TEETH

- Have person bite down on a rolled sterile dressing in the space left by the tooth
- Save any displaced teeth. Place them in milk, if possible, or water. Pick the tooth up by the crown (white part), not the root
- Call your dentist immediately for instructions on further care

ABDOMINAL INJURY

- Keep person lying down with knees bent, if possible

If organs are exposed:

- Do not apply pressure to organs or push back inside
- Remove any clothing from around wound
- Apply moist, sterile dressings or clean cloth loosely over wound
- Keep dressing moist with warm water
- Place a cloth over dressing to keep organs warm

WOUNDS — SPECIAL SITUATIONS

INFECTION

Germs can enter the body through scrapes, cuts, or punctures and cause infection. Infection can develop within hours or days of an injury.

SIGNALS

- Wound area becomes swollen and red
- Area may feel warm or throb with pain; may discharge pus
- Red streaks may develop around the wound
- Person may develop fever and feel ill

CARE

- Wash hands before and after caring for wound, even if you wear disposable gloves
- Wash minor wounds with soap and water
- Do not wash wounds that require medical attention unless instructed to do so by your health care provider
- Cover wound with clean dressing and bandage, change daily
- If infection persists or worsens, seek medical help

APPENDICES —

FIRST AID KIT

Be prepared for an emergency. Keep a first aid kit in your home and in your automobile. Carry a first aid kit with you or know where you can find one when you are participating in outdoor activities. Know the location of first aid kits where you work.

A first aid kit should include the following:

- Flashlight and batteries
- Scissors and tweezers
- Emergency blanket
- Triangular bandages
- Antiseptic towelettes
- Adhesive bandage strips in assorted sizes
- Gauze pads
- Roller gauze
- Adhesive tape
- Antiseptic ointment
- Disposable gloves
- Plastic bags
- Cold pack
- Breathing barrier
- Activated charcoal

This booklet is not a substitute for materials used in American Red Cross courses in which First Aid or CPR certification is given.

FIRST AID KIT

Whether you buy a first aid kit or put one together, make sure it has all the items you may need. Include a list of emergency phone numbers. Check the kit regularly to make sure flashlight batteries still work and that it contains all the necessary supplies. Replace any items that have expired. Keep a copy of *First Aid Fast* in your kit.

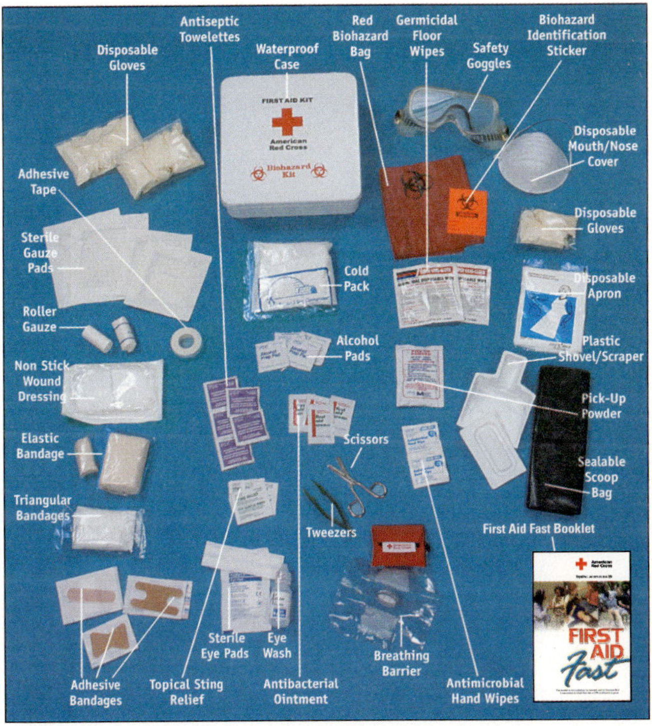

LIFE-SAVING SKILL SUMMARY

SKILL	ADULT (9 YEARS AND OLDER)
Rescue breathing (No breathing, shows movement in response to rescue breaths)	Give 1 slow breath about every 5 seconds; about 2 seconds per breath; 1 minute = about 12 breaths
Choking, conscious (Cannot cough, speak, or breathe)	Determine if person is choking; stand behind person and deliver abdominal thrusts; repeat until object is removed or victim loses consciousness
Choking, unconscious (Breaths do not go in)	Give 2 slow breaths; reposition airway and reattempt 2 slow breaths; if breaths do not go in, give 15 chest compressions; lift lower jaw and tongue; look in mouth and remove object if seen; give 2 slow breaths. Repeat 15 chest compressions, object look/removal, and 2 slow breaths until breaths go in, victim starts breathing, or EMS personnel arrive and take over
CPR (No breathing, no movement in response to rescue breaths)	Depth of compression is about 2 inches; compressions are performed with both hands; complete 15 compressions in about 10 seconds; do cycles of 15 compressions and 2 breaths

This booklet is not a substitute for materials used in American Red Cross courses in which First Aid or CPR certification is given.

LIFE-SAVING SKILL SUMMARY

CHILD (1 TO 8 YEARS)	INFANT (BIRTH TO 1 YEAR)
Give 1 slow breath about every 3 seconds; about 1½ seconds per breath; 1 minute = about 20 breaths	Give 1 slow breath about every 3 seconds; about 1½ seconds per breath; 1 minute = about 20 breaths
Determine if the child is choking; stand or kneel behind child and deliver abdominal thrusts; repeat until object is removed or child loses consciousness	Determine if infant is choking; give 5 back blows; give 5 chest thrusts; repeat until object is removed or infant loses consciousness
Give 2 slow breaths; reposition airway and reattempt 2 slow breaths; if breaths do not go in, give 5 chest compressions; lift lower jaw and tongue; look in mouth and remove object if seen; give 1 slow breath. Repeat 5 chest compressions, object look/removal, and 1 slow breath until breaths go in, victim starts breathing, or EMS personnel arrive and take over	Give 2 slow breaths; reposition airway and reattempt 2 slow breaths; if breaths do not go in, give 5 chest compressions; lift lower jaw and tongue; look in mouth and remove object if seen; give 1 slow breath. Repeat 5 chest compressions, object look/removal, and 1 slow breath until breaths go in, victim starts breathing, or EMS personnel arrive and take over
Depth of compression is about 1½ inches; compressions are performed with 1 hand; complete 5 compressions in about 3 seconds; do cycles of 5 compressions and 1 breath	Depth of compression is about 1 inch; compressions are performed with 2 fingers; complete 5 compressions in slightly less than 3 seconds; do cycles of 5 compressions and 1 breath

HOW AND WHEN TO CALL 9-1-1

CALL 9-1-1 OR THE LOCAL EMERGENCY NUMBER IF SOMEONE

- Is or becomes unconscious
- Has trouble breathing or is breathing in a strange way
- Has chest pain or pressure
- Is bleeding severely
- Has pressure or pain in the abdomen that does not go away
- Is vomiting or passing blood
- Has seizures, a severe headache, or slurred speech
- Appears to have been poisoned
- Has injuries to the head, neck, or back
- Has possible broken bones

BE PREPARED TO GIVE

- Location (street address, city or town, cross streets, landmarks, etc.)
- Phone number from where you are calling
- Your name
- What happened
- How many injured
- Conditions of person(s) requiring aid
- Help (CARE) being given

Do not hang up first. Let the dispatcher hang up first.

This booklet is not a substitute for materials used in American Red Cross courses in which First Aid or CPR certification is given.

HOW AND WHEN TO CALL 9-1-1

WHEN YOU ARE ALONE

Call FIRST for:

- An unconscious adult or child 8 years old or older
- An unconscious infant or child known to be at high risk for heart problems

Call FAST, after providing one minute of care, for:

- An unconscious victim less than 8 years old
- Any victim of submersion or near drowning
- Any victim of cardiac arrest associated with trauma
- Any victim of drug overdose

EMERGENCY PHONE NUMBERS

LOCAL EMERGENCY NUMBER

POISON CONTROL CENTER

FIRE

POLICE

DOCTORS

OTHER IMPORTANT NUMBERS

This booklet is not a substitute for materials used in American Red Cross courses in which First Aid or CPR certification is given.